The Athlete's Guide to CBD

The Athlete's Guide to *CBD*

Treat Pain and Inflammation,
Maximize Recovery,
and Sleep Better Naturally

Scott Douglas

Foreword by Tiki Barber

RODALE.

NEW YORK

Copyright © 2019 by Scott Douglas

All rights reserved.
Published in the United States by Rodale Books, an imprint of Random House, a division of Penguin Random House LLC, New York.
rodalebooks.com

RODALE and the Plant colophon are registered trademarks of Penguin Random House LLC.

Library of Congress Cataloging-in-Publication Data is available upon request.

ISBN 978-0-593-13580-8
Ebook ISBN 978-0-593-13581-5

Printed in the United States of America

Book design by Patrice Sheridan
Cover design by Pete Garceau

10 9 8 7 6 5 4 3 2 1

First Edition

Contents

Foreword

As a former player in the National Football League and current radio and television sports broadcaster, I've gotten used to hearing about cannabis by the subtle, yet obvious phrasing used by the league when disciplining its players. "XYZ athlete has been suspended for violation of the league's policy for substances of abuse" is a typical statement. This policy, not to be confused with the NFL's policy for performance-enhancing drugs, is likely rooted in the federal government's classification of cannabis as a Schedule 1 drug under the guidelines of the Drug Enforcement Agency, which means that they view cannabis as potentially addictive and providing absolutely no medical value.

Clearly, that assessment is flawed and narrow-minded. The stigma around cannabis is preventing people from realizing some amazing benefits. And CBD, which doesn't get you high and is derived from hemp, not cannabis, is often caught in the crossfire. The anecdotal evidence is strong, and as the tide toward decriminalization and legalization of cannabis continues around the world, we will hopefully see more clinical studies that support what cancer patients, anxiety sufferers, and the countless folks who use cannabis and CBD to manage pain have been swearing by for years.

I believe in the healing properties of CBD and cannabis so much that I cofounded an investment firm that aims to bring sophisticated financing, technology, and marketing execution to the cannabis business, hopefully advancing developments in the industry worldwide. Personally, I've found that CBD helps with my athletic performance, and I believe that it has the potential to be a major asset to the athletic community.

Scott Douglas's new book, *The Athlete's Guide to CBD*, reaffirms that belief. It is one of the most interesting and informative guides to delve into the topic—not only does it provide a backstory about the ever-evolving world of CBD, it also gives a layman's understanding of the complexities surrounding use by those of us who consider ourselves athletes.

Whether you're a professional who's looking for a way to manage the rigors of a long season, a weekend warrior trying to best his neighborhood peers, or simply a health-conscious individual looking to find the right balance in your life, understanding the function and benefits of CBD can be eye-opening.

—Tiki Barber,
former NFL Pro Bowl player; cofounder of Grover Group Management,
a global management and consulting firm for the cannabis industry;
and TV personality and CBS Sports Radio host

Introduction

CBD has officially gone mainstream. And with widespread claims that the nonintoxicating cannabis product can reduce inflammation and pain, improve sleep and mental focus, and restore overall balance to the body naturally, CBD has piqued the interest of athletes.

Don't let the word *athlete* in this book's title intimidate you. Athletes aren't just those in professional or school sports. Athletes are people who work out with purpose. That purpose can be to compete, to perform better than you have before, to add years to your life, to add life to your years, or any combination of these and other reasons. If you exercise regularly and care about your workouts, you're an athlete.

I consider myself one such person. I started running as a teenager in 1979. I've run almost every day since, and when I've had a running injury I've usually done some other type of daily workout. (I'm the sort who was doing a lot of cycling while waiting for one running injury to heal, so figured I might as well ride a century.) I've run races as short as 100 meters and as long as 50 kilometers. I've also had years when I ran no races but considered myself as much of an athlete as when I could run at a sub-5:00 mile pace for 10 kilometers.

Since the early 1990s, I've been fortunate enough to combine my athletic interests with my professional ones. I've held senior editorial positions at *Runner's World* and the late, lamented *Running Times*. I've written and cowritten several running books and have written about broader health and fitness topics for publications such as the *Washington Post, The Atlantic,* and *Slate.*

Being a veteran in both sports and journalism is pertinent to this book. My profession encourages healthy skepticism. So does running. Any intellectually honest athlete knows there are no magic bullets, cure-alls, or "secrets." Hard work, dedication, and consistency are the keys to success.

At the same time, successful athletes are open-minded. Training methods, gear, and sports nutrition are vastly more sophisticated than they were a century ago. So obviously, there have to be some new ideas and products worth testing. Many of us are willing to try something different if we think the underlying rationale seems sound. Then we'll run it through the ultimate lab of daily training and see if it helps some aspect of our athletic life. Most of the time, the answer is no. You don't hear much about the barefoot-style, gloves-for-your-toes minimalist running shoes these days, and it's been decades since lots of athletes gobbled down salt tablets and bee pollen.

So when I started adding CBD to my routine in the spring of 2018, I did so with foundational skepticism. But I was also open to the idea that it could be one of the rare new offerings worth incorporating into my regimen. I pretty quickly concluded the answer was yes. As I'll describe later,

I feel that CBD improves my sleep, speeds my recovery from training, and helps me to manage athletic injuries, some minor, some more significant. These benefits mean that I enjoy my running—and my life—more.

Many of my running friends have since investigated CBD for themselves. They know I'm not a bandwagon jumper or susceptible to snake oil sales pitches. They've asked me about my experiences with CBD and the underlying ideas about how it might help improve our athletic lives.

My goal in this book is to have that conversation with you. Pretend we're working out together. You're curious about whether CBD can help you as an athlete, and you heard I've been looking into the matter. I start by covering the basics—what CBD is, how it works, how much to take, what to look for when shopping. Then I go into more detail on the things that could be of special benefit to us athletes, like managing injuries, recovering faster, and sleeping better.

What I tell you is informed by talking with other athletes who use CBD, sports medicine professionals who've incorporated it into their practices, industry insiders and other experts in the field, relevant research, and, where appropriate, my own experiences. What I share is also informed by the healthy skepticism you'd want from anyone suggesting you try something new. I encourage you to view CBD not as a cure-all—we both know better than that—but as a helpful addition that can multiply the benefits of other good athletic practices.

By the end, you'll know enough to smartly conduct your own CBD experiment. And for quick reference, you'll find a glossary of CBD-related terms and a buyer's checklist at the back of this book.

Chapter 1

An Overview of CBD

Diving into the world of CBD can be overwhelming. The first step is understanding the basics—what CBD is, what it does, how it works. That's what this chapter is about.

CBD is shorthand for *cannabidiol*. It's one of the more than 100 cannabinoids—chemical compounds that act on receptors in your body—found in the cannabis plant.

CBD and tetrahydrocannabinol (THC) are the two most prevalent cannabinoids in the cannabis plant. THC is the cannabinoid that produces a marijuana high. CBD won't get you high. It's often said to be "nonpsychoactive," but that description is inaccurate. Because CBD can reduce anxiety and depression, and improve mood and mental acuity, it does have psychological effects. It's more accurate to say that CBD is nonintoxicating.

CBD and THC are two different varieties of the same plant, *Cannabis sativa*. The key factor in whether that plant is called marijuana or hemp is how much THC it contains. Hemp is a cannabis plant that contains less than 0.3 percent THC. Marijuana contains more than that amount of THC.

If it seems confusing that marijuana and hemp are the same species of plant, think about tomatoes. The species name for cherry tomatoes and beefsteak tomatoes is *Solanum lycopersicum,* even though they look and taste quite different. There can be great variety within one species.

Marijuana can also contain large amounts of CBD, depending on its strain and cultivation. Medical marijuana often contains a relatively high concentration of CBD to temper the intoxicating effects of THC. There are indications from some studies that the combination of THC and CBD can be more effective for some medical conditions than either of the cannabinoids alone.

Of course, in the United States, marijuana is illegal at the federal level and is legalized for recreational use in only 10 states and the District of Columbia. So almost all mass-market CBD products are made from hemp, not marijuana. In this book, we'll consider only hemp-derived CBD products (i.e., nonintoxicating ones).

In most cases, when people say they're taking CBD they mean a product of which CBD extracted from hemp is one ingredient. For efficiency's sake, I'll do the same. The most popular CBD product types include oil-based tinctures, capsules, and topical solutions (meant to be applied to your skin rather than swallowed). We'll look in detail at the various product types and how to take them in the next chapter.

What Is CBD Said to Do?

Maybe a better question is: What *isn't* CBD said to do?

Depending on whom you listen to, CBD is said to help treat epilepsy, cancer, Parkinson's disease, Alzheimer's disease, other neurodegenerative diseases, cerebral ischemia, diabetes, rheumatoid arthritis, osteoarthritis, inflammatory bowel disease, other inflammatory diseases, nausea, neuropathic pain, anxiety, depression, schizophrenia, insomnia, drug addiction, and many other conditions.

So far, the evidence for many of these claims is anecdotal rather than clinical. One exception is Epidiolex, the first CBD medication approved by the Food and Drug Administration. It's an oral solution prescribed to treat seizures associated with two rare and severe forms of epilepsy, Lennox–Gastaut syndrome and Dravet syndrome, in patients age two and older. Epidiolex is an isolate form of CBD derived from marijuana.

Otherwise, the FDA doesn't allow medical claims for CBD. Manufacturers can't promise their products will diagnose, treat, or cure diseases. That's why CBD product literature contains broad phrases like "restore vitality," "relax and recover," and "may keep healthy people healthy."

The FDA is famously, and probably laudably, conservative in this regard. Scientists also tend toward conservatism in discussing cause and effect. Still, those investigating CBD are willing to write in peer-reviewed journals things like this sentence from *Pharmacotherapy:* "CBD exhibits neuroprotective, antiepileptic, anxiolytic [antianxiety], antipsychotic, and anti-inflammatory properties." In this book, we'll focus on the claims for CBD that have the most relevance for athletes and a decent amount of support behind them.

Is CBD Legal?

The short answer is that you the consumer can legally buy hemp-derived CBD throughout the United States. That includes buying it online. The longer answer is that there remains legal murkiness around CBD, more on technical grounds than in practical terms. So to reiterate: If you want to buy hemp-derived CBD, you may with no fear of getting arrested. If that answer satisfies you, feel free to skip the following more detailed explanation.

CBD started to take off commercially only after the passage of the 2014 federal farm bill. That legislation allowed for the cultivation and marketing of hemp if those activities were for research purposes; were part of an agricultural pilot program or other agricultural or academic program; and were permitted by state laws. The farm bill excluded hemp grown under those conditions from the long-standing federal classification of hemp as a Schedule 1 controlled substance, the same classification given to marijuana. Federal law prohibits commercial production and sale of Schedule 1 substances.

In 2016, the US Department of Agriculture, the Drug Enforcement Administration, and the Food and Drug Administration issued guidance on the sale of products made from hemp grown under the provisions of the 2014 farm bill. The guidance said that these products—read: hemp-derived CBD—could be sold for "purposes of marketing research" but "not for the purpose of general commercial activity."

If that sounds confusing, it is. People who started a CBD business after the 2014 farm bill became law could have argued that they were conducting "marketing research" on such products, just to gather information on whether and how people might be interested in CBD tinctures. Would that argument hold up in court? Who knows? Also, many said that the "not for the purpose of general commercial activity" phrase went against the intent of the 2014 farm bill. Adding to the uncertainty was that guidance of the sort released in 2016 isn't legally binding.

But wait, there's more! In 2018, a rider to a federal appropriations act prohibited federal agencies from using federal money in conflict with the 2014 farm bill. That rider included the processing and sale of hemp grown under the farm bill regulations, inside or outside the state in which it was grown. These clauses were widely taken to mean that the federal government was going to let the CBD market be.

"It was a ridiculous situation when operating under the 2014 farm bill," says Tom Adams, managing director and principal analyst for the consumer cannabis research firm BDS Analytics. "There was language with a loophole big enough to drive a truck full of CBD through, and everybody did."

When enacted, the 2014 farm bill's provisions were to be in place for four years. The 2018 farm bill, signed into law with just a few days remaining in the year, did as expected: it legalized hemp at the federal level. That change was anticipated and celebrated by the CBD industry. Legalization removed whatever concern remained about running afoul of federal drug laws and is widely expected to lead to far more hemp cultivation. And yet . . .

The farm bill legalized hemp. That's not the same as saying that products made from hemp aren't subject to federal scrutiny. Within hours of hemp's legalization, the FDA released a statement about CBD. The gist was that, because of its approval of Epidiolex, the FDA considers CBD to be a drug, not a food additive approved for interstate commerce. Parsing this decree means that the FDA views some CBD products (oils, capsules, and other types that are digested) differently than others (vaping, topical balms, and other types that your body doesn't process like food).

So uncertainty for the CBD industry remains. "Everyone's still operating in that gray area much like they were before," says Riley Cote, owner of BodyChek Wellness. "But until they make a case of someone and shut them down or send notices, we'll keep operating as we have. Nobody's going to slow down. In fact, everyone's ramping up."

We'll look at this latest wrinkle in more detail in the final chapter. For now, the answer to the is-it-legal question remains as I stated above: you, the consumer, will not be arrested for buying hemp-derived CBD products.

Is CBD Safe?

"The first question I always get is, 'Will this get me high?'" Skyler Bissell, CEO of the CBD powder company Oleo, says. "The second is, 'Will it hurt me?'" We've already covered that the answer to the first question is no. The answer to the second question also appears to be overwhelmingly no.

Hector Lopez, MD, helped to start a company called Supplement Safety Solutions, which helps supplement makers monitor and report adverse reactions to their products. "For CBD, there have been no significant adverse reactions reported in more than one million doses sold," he says. "I would say CBD's safety profile is remarkably high."

In 2011, Brazilian researchers published a review of studies on CBD in the journal *Current Drug Safety*. They concluded that CBD appears to have few undesirable side effects. It doesn't affect appetite, heart rate, body temperature, blood pressure, or fine motor skills. The researchers also concluded that chronic use and doses up to 1,500 milligrams a day appear to be well tolerated. (For comparison's sake, most people taking CBD consume less than 50 milligrams a day.) As we'll see in the next chapter, the main reported side effects are drowsiness, fatigue, and diarrhea. These usually happen when you take too much CBD, and they dissipate or disappear when you reduce your dosage. A follow-up review, published in *Cannabis and Cannabinoid Research* in 2017, confirmed the earlier findings.

The primary cautionary note for most people has to do with drug interactions. CBD is heavily metabolized by the liver. It's possible that CBD's interactions with enzymes in the liver could affect how the liver metabolizes a second substance, such as a prescription medication. Depending on the nature of the chemical interaction, more of the prescription medication might get metabolized in the presence of CBD, or less might get metabolized.

CBD has been postulated to affect the absorption of some blood thinners and antidepressants. Drug interactions of any sort can be extraordinarily complex. A quick tip is that CBD appears to interact with medications in the same way that grapefruit juice does but perhaps more potently. If you've been told to watch your grapefruit intake while on a certain medication, it's a good idea to ask your doctor about taking CBD while on that drug.

How Does CBD Work?

Understanding how CBD produces its potential benefits starts with, interestingly enough, marijuana.

The cannabis plant has been used to treat pain and other ailments for centuries. As with many traditional medicine practices, people didn't know why cannabis seemed to work. They just knew that it helped them feel better. In the twentieth century, scientists started looking for answers. They were primarily interested in why marijuana produces the subjective feeling of a high, but they also wanted to learn how it provides pain relief and other benefits. In 1964, THC was identified as the intoxicating agent in marijuana. But how exactly THC produced its effects remained unknown.

The answer came in 1988 with the discovery of receptors in the body that THC binds to. THC activates these receptors, which are located on the surface of cells throughout the body. These were named cannabinoid receptors. Within a few years, two main types of cannabinoid receptors, CB1 and CB2, were distinguished. CB1 receptors are located primarily in nerve cells in the brain and spinal cord, while CB2 receptors can be found in the immune and gastrointestinal systems.

If the body has receptors for cannabinoids, then shouldn't

the body have its own cannabinoids? It does, and they were discovered a few years after the receptors were identified.

"We produce molecules in the body called endocannabinoids, which bind and activate cannabinoid receptors located on cells throughout the body," says Nicholas DiPatrizio, PhD, a professor of biomedical sciences at the University of California, Riverside School of Medicine. "Think of endocannabinoids as our body's natural cannabis, in that THC hijacks and activates the same receptors as do endocannabinoids." ("Endo" means "produced from within.") The two types of endocannabinoids are anandamide and 2-arachidonoylglycerol (2-AG). DiPatrizio uses the analogy of locks and keys to help nonscientists visualize the interaction of receptors and cannabinoids (either endocannabinoids or external cannabinoids, especially THC). Receptors are the locks and cannabinoids are the keys. When cannabinoids "unlock" the receptors, cellular changes occur in the organ associated with the receptors.

Together, endocannabinoids and cannabinoid receptors are called the endocannabinoid system. Once scientists understood the system's basic structure, subsequent research led to understanding its profound importance. "The endocannabinoid system is found in every organ throughout the body and controls many physiological processes, including food intake and energy balance, learning and memory, and pain processing, to name a few," DiPatrizio says. "It's located everywhere and it's involved in regulating almost every physiological function that scientists study."

In this view, the endocannabinoid system is often called things like the body's "master regulator" or "control system" and is said to be responsible for maintaining homeostasis, or stable equilibrium among other bodily systems. The endo-cannabinoid system becomes upregulated, which is to say more active, when the body is under physical and/or psychological stress.

What does this have to do with CBD? The basic idea is that, as a cannabinoid, CBD can act upon the endocannabinoid system and improve its functioning. Improve the endocannabinoid system's functioning, and you theoretically improve key bodily functions. Hence the vast potential benefits claimed for CBD.

The precise mechanism by which CBD acts upon the endocannabinoid system hasn't been delineated. It doesn't appear to bind to CB1 and CB2 receptors as strongly as THC does. But with CBD being nonintoxicating, it's possible to take relatively high doses to increase activation of those receptors. "It's unclear whether CBD directly affects the CB1 and CB2 receptors or if there's more of a subtle interplay with the body," says Scott Palmer, MD, a team physician for the Chicago White Sox and Chicago Bulls. "We're still figuring this out."

One example of that subtle interplay is CBD reducing the breakdown of or improving signaling of anandamide, one of the two endocannabinoids. The word *anandamide* is derived from the Sanskrit word *ananda,* meaning "bliss" or "joy." Higher levels of anandamide are thought to contribute to the feelings of euphoria many people have during and after exercise. Palmer says that CBD can stimulate the same neurotransmitters targeted by modern antidepressant medications and can block the same pain receptors that common anti-inflammatory drugs do.

This all sounds pretty good! But one night, when

my inner skeptic was working overtime, I woke with the thought: Dogs and other mammals have endocannabinoid systems; biologically, it's been around forever. So if the endocannabinoid system is so important, why does it need an outside product, and an expensive one at that, to function optimally? Why didn't we evolve with a self-sufficient endocannabinoid system?

The executive summary of the answer I got: the endocannabinoid system didn't evolve in athletes living in twenty-first-century Western society.

"When the endocannabinoid system becomes really active is when it's under challenge," DiPatrizio says. "Most research looks at the body under a pathological challenge, like a metabolic challenge such as diet-induced diabetes. But I think you can infer that modern life, or hard athletic training, could cause the system to become overactive."

David Raichlen, PhD, a professor of anthropology at the University of Arizona who has studied the endocannabinoid system and exercise, says, "It doesn't need something [external], but that doesn't necessarily mean we can't find ways to piggyback on natural systems and enhance the effects."

These are reasonable answers, and it should be said that DiPatrizio and Raichlen make these pro-CBD points even though neither feels a personal need to take CBD. Some of Raichlen's research has been on the energy expenditure of the Hadza people, who are hunter-gatherers in northern Tanzania. In one study, he found that a typical Hadza man covers about seven miles a day by foot. That level of activity is probably similar to how our long-ago ancestors lived. But the Hadza cover that distance mostly at a leisurely pace, and the work is spread throughout the day. That's a different undertaking than getting up while it's dark and squeezing in a seven-mile run on asphalt before you get the kids ready for school and rush off to work.

What Does Research on CBD Show?

"Extraordinary claims require extraordinary evidence," DiPatrizio says. To date, there's little of what he and other scientists would consider "extraordinary evidence" for many of CBD's purported benefits, at least in the form of large clinical trials on humans. In Chapters 4 through 7, we'll look at what research shows about CBD and specific aspects of being an athlete. For now, let's look at the overall state of CBD research.

It helps to bear in mind how scientific research on humans is done. The parameters of research are as tight as possible. The study's aim should be well defined: Does a specific intervention (such as a medication) improve a specific condition (such as incidence of epileptic seizures)? The participants should be divided into two otherwise identical groups, half of whom receive the intervention and half of whom receive what should be a noneffective intervention, or placebo (the classic "sugar pill" in medication trials). Neither the subjects nor the researchers should know who is getting the "real" intervention, on the theory that knowing who's getting what can skew the results. Another ideal is specificity in the intervention—for example, pill X has this precise chemical structure and was of this precise potency throughout the study. At the end of the trial period, results are analyzed to see if the group receiving the intervention improved more than the control group. Again, this is the ideal.

Perhaps you've already guessed one reason why CBD research can be problematic. To have as few variables as possible, it makes sense to use a CBD isolate in a study. That way, if you find the intervention works, you can more safely conclude that this specific CBD product was responsible. In the real world, however, when most people talk about CBD's effectiveness, they're talking about what are called full-spectrum products, which contain not just CBD but other parts of the hemp plant. So if you get good results from a full-spectrum product, is it the CBD or something else? Also, those products can vary greatly, owing to factors such as the soil the hemp was grown in and the weather while the plant was grown. A whole plant's heterogeneous nature makes replicating one study's findings in subsequent studies more difficult. Think of this as the difference between research on a chemical isolate of vitamin C and research on oranges.

Further muddying things is that a fair amount of research has looked at cannabis solutions that include THC and CBD, because of the aforementioned evidence that the two cannabinoids together are more effective at addressing many conditions. Much of that research was spurred by the widespread use of cannabis to self-treat pain, insomnia, and other conditions. "CBD was isolated and identified before THC," Karyemaitre Aliffe, MD, a longtime researcher and proponent of medical cannabis, says. "But research on CBD wasn't carried forward because what people were interested in was what gets you high. CBD resumed being in the spotlight only recently because as people accept that cannabis is good for pain, good for insomnia, some say, 'Yes, but it makes you high—that's terrible. So let's go back and look at CBD.'"

In doing this type of research, you also want to study as specific an outcome as possible. That laser focus existed in the Epidiolex trials. It's easy to record that a child went from having 20 seizures a day to 4 after taking CBD. The same is true of research suggesting reduced spasticity in people with multiple sclerosis. But think about why most people take CBD—to sleep better, to be less anxious, to have less pain. These outcomes can be measured, but they're broader and less quantifiably straightforward.

Much of the research on CBD and cannabinoids in general has been done outside of the United States; Israel and Canada have been among the leaders. That's largely because of past US regulatory issues over marijuana and hemp. Science is science regardless of geography. But human clinical trials are expensive, and not all places have the resources available to US laboratories. Most CBD research has been preclinical, which is to say on animals (usually rodents). "Preclinical studies point very strongly to huge potential for CBD across the board of human conditions," Philip Blair, MD, says. Tim Drennan, who develops CBD products for several brands, including his own, MYKU Wellness, says about rodent studies, "[They've] proven to be a very good way to establish proof of concept, that this is something that merits further research. But is it worth it to then fund human trials? That's where we hit a barrier."

The CBD industry has funded little meaningful research because of the cost. A small observational study conducted by a physician, in which people with a condition are given a treatment and followed over time, can cost $3 to $5 million. "That's not going to get you FDA approval," Drennan says. "You can say we funded this study and got these results, but that's it. For a lot of us it's more effective to focus on making effective products and letting people find out for themselves if they work."

Large clinical trials of the sort that would garner FDA approval cost magnitudes more. Only large pharmaceutical companies have the resources to fund those. But do they have the incentive? As a product of nature, CBD is considered in the public domain and can't be patented. What can be patented are the processes leading to production and the methods of use. That's how GW Pharmaceuticals patented its CBD-isolate product Epidiolex. Future CBD-related patents are likely to be around other specific disease states. That approach makes financial sense, and of course there's a great public health value in discovering new ways to treat disease. But findings in that vein are far afield from clinical research on the broad matters of health, wellness, and performance that most CBD users have a personal stake in.

The current status of research on CBD need not be a deal breaker, especially for athletes. After all, there are many things we do, such as stretching after workouts or strengthening our core muscles, that haven't been "proven" by peer-reviewed clinical research but that most of us find helpful. In other cases, science eventually gets around to explaining some of the why behind what athletes have discovered for themselves, such as interval training and eating a high-carbohydrate diet in the few days before a long race.

CBD's Status in the Medical Community

To date, most people taking CBD have learned about it from sources other than medical professionals. In one survey of CBD consumers, 75 percent said that family, friends, or the internet was their primary source of information, and only 10 percent learned about CBD from their doctor. Why aren't more physicians discussing CBD with their patients?

Part of the explanation is the current state of research on CBD. As we saw, research has mostly looked at CBD in isolate form as a treatment for specific medical conditions. FDA approval of Epidiolex should spur research on additional conditions, especially after the federal legalization of hemp. But those studies are still pretty far removed from whether a dropper of CBD before bed every night might enhance your overall recovery from athletic training. "They're looking for the double-blind, controlled clinical studies to prove that it's effective," Blair says of his fellow physicians who are skeptical. "I appreciate that, but those studies are years in the making, and there's quite a bit of variability in the products available." Reinforcing this point about variability in CBD, Aliffe says, "Pharmacology is linear—a single drug having a single action and a singular effect. To believe that, you have to ignore a lot of other things and call them side effects. As soon as you go from a single purified molecule like CBD to a whole plant like cannabis, you suddenly have diverse, systemic effects."

Of course, we all want to be treated by a doctor who has done her homework. Evidence-based modern medicine is to be treasured. At the same time, doctors don't consistently apply this thinking about lack of clinical evidence. "Physicians seem to hold CBD to a different standard, when they're using a number of different drugs and procedures that are not FDA-approved," Blair says. For example, it's estimated that more than half of antidepressant prescriptions in the United States are off-label—in other words, they're for conditions other than what the drugs were approved to treat.

Medical school might perpetuate the atomistic view of patient care that Aliffe and others find dissatisfying. From a realm that we athletes can appreciate, a study of med school criteria found that only 18 percent of schools required a class on physical activity and that fewer than half included any courses on exercise. This is despite the overwhelming evidence that regular exercise improves almost all aspects of health. Blair, a former army physician, says that the endocannabinoid system is taught at only a few medical schools. "There's no awareness that we have this pervasive system throughout our bodies that has a great deal to do with homeostasis and balancing out so many other systems," he says.

Palmer and his fellow pro sports team physician Charles Bush-Joseph, MD, are more optimistic. Palmer says that he's seen a great increase in interest in CBD among his peers the past few years. "Some MDs may be unaware of what's going on specifically scientifically, but I think everybody is open to using it," he says. Bush-Joseph notes that many young physicians are looking for nontraditional and natural treatment options for their patients. CBD might be an instance of patients educating doctors, not vice versa.

Who Is Taking CBD?

Two fairly large surveys give some insight into the demographics of CBD. (As with any survey, the results are subject to who participates.) One was conducted by a cannabis company, HelloMD, and a cannabis industry analysis firm, the Brightfield Group, in 2017. Of the 2,400 HelloMD customers who participated, 59 percent were women. The age group with the highest representation was ages 35 to 49 (31 percent of respondents), followed by 50 to 59 and 22 to 34 (22 percent for both groups). The top conditions these CBD users were attempting to address were anxiety, insomnia, joint pain and inflammation, depression, muscle tension or strain, and severe or chronic pain.

Another survey of 2,400 CBD users, published in *Cannabis and Cannabinoid Research* in 2018, produced similar results. Women constituted 52 percent of respondents. The age group with the largest representation was ages 55 to 64 (24 percent), followed by 45 to 54 and 35 to 44 (both 18 percent). Perhaps reflecting the cost of CBD, 71 percent of respondents were in college, were college graduates, or held an advanced degree.

Almost two-thirds (62 percent) said they used CBD for a medical condition. The top conditions cited were chronic pain, arthritis/joint pain, anxiety, depression, and insomnia or sleep disorder. Of this subgroup, 36 percent said CBD alone worked well enough to manage their condition. Just over one-third (38 percent) said they used CBD primarily for general health and well-being. Almost half (48 percent) of both groups said they took CBD daily and that, at the time of the survey, they'd been taking it for less than a year.

Residents from all US states were represented in the 2018 survey. Anecdotally, there's geographic variance among CBD users. "You go somewhere like New York City and see it in gyms, stores, lots of places," says Michael Tatz, founder of the athlete-focused brand Resilience. "Most other parts of the country there's not that level of permeation yet."

Is It Okay for Athletes to Take CBD?

In the athletic world, CBD was removed from the World Anti-Doping Agency's list of prohibited substances in 2018. The World Anti-Doping Agency is the organization that creates and enforces rules on performance-enhancing drugs for competitive athletes and that regulates Olympic conduct. This action doesn't necessarily mean that CBD has no benefit for athletes. Many things that can improve performance aren't on WADA's prohibited list, such as sports drinks and lighter bikes. A substance goes on WADA's list if it meets at least two of these three criteria:

- It has the potential to improve athletic performance.
- It carries at least a theoretical health risk.
- It violates the spirit of sport.

So while sports drinks and CBD have the potential to improve performance, they're not a health risk when used as indicated, and they don't violate the spirit of sport (in part because they're readily available to all competitors).

The US Anti-Doping Agency is responsible for enforcing the WADA code in the United States. The USADA notes that, although CBD is permitted, all other cannabinoids, including THC, remain prohibited in competition. There are two takeaways from that message.

First, "in competition" refers to doping tests administered on the day of competition. Some substances are allowed during training but are prohibited in competition. For example, beta-blockers are prohibited in competition in sports such as archery, golf, and darts (!) because they can reduce tremor. In contrast, EPO, which boosts red blood cell production, is prohibited at all times, because taking it during a training block can enable workouts that would otherwise not be possible. So having any trace of THC or other cannabinoids besides CBD in your blood or urine can make you fail a postrace doping test.

Second, and related, the USADA warns athletes that CBD in its most popular forms contains other cannabinoids. Again, hemp is defined as containing not more than 0.3 percent THC. But trace amounts of THC are possible, USADA warns, especially given studies that have found discrepancies between the claimed contents and the actual contents of some CBD products. (We'll look at this issue in Chapter 3.) CBD isolates are available but might nonetheless contain other cannabinoids, the USADA says. Between that uncertainty and the possibility of cannabinoids staying in the body long after they're taken, the overall message from the USADA to elite athletes subject to drug testing is: be careful with CBD.

CBD's status in college athletics and major professional sports leagues is murkier. The NCAA's prohibited-substances list includes marijuana but not CBD. But the list says that substances that are "chemically related" to prohibited substances are also banned. This was presumably why, in 2018, Auburn University told a promising high school football player, C. J. Harris, that he couldn't play in college if he continued taking CBD for his epileptic seizures. The National Football League and National Basketball Association prohibit cannabis and don't distinguish between marijuana and hemp.

"Athletes will say, 'Someone gave me CBD but I don't

dare use it, because what if it gives me a false positive for THC on a drug test?'" Palmer says.

This uncertainty—and lack of knowledge—is one reason why you don't yet see scores of pro athletes touting CBD on television. (Another is probably a lack of sponsorship deals, given that most CBD companies are small businesses.) "Once people get an understanding, I think CBD will have a role in professional sports," Palmer says.

Few of us, of course, are subject to athletic doping tests or eligible for professional contracts. But it's nice to know that CBD is an allowed substance in worldwide sports and is approved by most US organizations and that using it doesn't violate the spirit of sport. So let's start looking at how taking it might help your workouts.

Key Points on an Overview of CBD

- CBD, or cannabidiol, is a component of the cannabis plant that may provide many health and athletic benefits.
- CBD is nonintoxicating, legal, and safe to take.
- CBD is thought to work by improving the functioning of the endocannabinoid system, which can be thought of as your body's master regulator.
- Forward-looking medical professionals increasingly embrace CBD's promise.

Chapter 2

How to Take CBD

Saying, "I'm going to start taking CBD" is a little like saying, "I'm going to start working out." What type of workout? Will you do more than one form of exercise? How often will you work out? How much will you exercise per session? How will you know that your workout is enough to be effective but not so much as to be deleterious?

Similarly, deciding to give CBD a go involves answering some basic questions—what form, how much, how often, and so on. In later chapters, we'll get into more detail on the best approach for specific goals, such as speeding recovery and improving sleep. For now, let's take an overview of the main consuming-CBD considerations. We'll start with the main product types for athletes.

Oils/Tinctures

This is probably what you have in mind when you think about CBD—the dark, tiny bottles with a dropper screwed into the top. Tinctures are the bestselling form of CBD, accounting for close to 40 percent of sales. A typical bottle contains 30 one-dropper servings.

Common descriptions include "CBD oil" and "hemp extract oil." Those phrases are a little misleading. When you buy something like olive oil or peanut oil, you're getting the oil of that plant. In this case, you're not getting the oil of cannabidiol; instead, the cannabidiol (and, usually, other parts of the hemp plant) have been mixed with a non-hemp form of oil. Medium-chain triglyceride oil, usually extracted from coconut oil, is the industry standard for the carrier agent of CBD. You might also see products simply called "hemp extract," with no mention of CBD or oil. For practical purposes, consider them the same as CBD oil and hemp extract oil.

To take this form of CBD, you squeeze the dropper to partly or completely fill it. Then you place the dropper under your tongue and squeeze the dropper to empty it. Taking a liquid this way is called "sublingual," meaning "under the tongue." The standard recommendation is to keep the oil under your tongue for 30 to 60 seconds before swallowing. Doing so allows some of it to be absorbed by the mucous membranes in your mouth. This type of absorption is said to result in more CBD being delivered throughout your body.

Taking CBD in this way can be a little odd at first, as the sublingual stall-then-swallow method isn't something that otherwise pops up in daily life. When I began taking a nightly dropper before bed, I often felt like I wound up with a mouthful of saliva while waiting the prescribed 30 to 60 seconds. I pictured the CBD oil running over the side of my teeth rather than being absorbed or, eventually, swallowed. Then I'd start worrying that I'd wasted the roughly two dollars' worth of oil I'd just put in my mouth. Not a great way to relax before sleep! I eventually got more adept, thanks mostly to swallowing any pooling saliva in my mouth before dipping into the tincture.

The taste of CBD oil varies widely, and does so independently of potency. I've had some fairly strong tinctures that are almost flavor-free, and I've had some normal-potency ones that taste the way I imagine a joint dipped in oil would. Most have at least a slight cannabis flavor. Some brands add natural flavoring, such as cinnamon or citron, which do a nice job of overriding most of the cannabis skunk taste (and odor). On the whole, CBD isolate oils have a milder flavor. (*Isolate* means that CBD is the only cannabinoid in the product. Contrast that with "broad-spectrum" or "full-spectrum" oils. We'll look at the touted benefit of full-spectrum products over isolates in the next chapter.) All, of course, have an oily feel while in your mouth.

A first cousin to tinctures are sprays. The idea here is to increase absorption by better penetrating the mucous membranes with smaller particles. Sprays are also a more familiar means of delivery for most people. The several I've tried had neither the pronounced cannabis taste nor the oily mouth feel of most tinctures. A potential drawback is less certainty about how much you're taking at once.

In all cases, be sure that you're buying a hemp extract containing CBD, not hemp seed oil. While the latter has its own healthful qualities, such as containing omega-3 fatty acids and essential amino acids, it doesn't contain cannabinoids, including CBD. What to look for when shopping is the subject of the next chapter; the quick takeaway here is to make sure the tincture or spray you're looking at says on the label how many milligrams of CBD it contains.

Capsules

I'm including soft gels, caplets, and similar items under the "capsule" umbrella. Think of these as the pill form of CBD.

The high-quality capsules you'll want to focus on as an athlete will contain just the ingredients needed to hold the product together, such as water, gelatin, and glycerin. Taste shouldn't be much of a consideration, because nearly all of the products are designed to be swallowed without chewing. (Chewable tablets are starting to come to market.) Some I've tried have a slight cannabis flavor on the way down. If, like me, you're the curious sort, and you break open capsules meant to be swallowed whole, prepare for any number of different tastes from the powder within, from nearly no flavor to tangy sweetness to a heavy earthiness.

Two big advantages of capsules are convenience and knowing exactly how much CBD you're consuming—any product in this vein worth taking will clearly state how much CBD is in each capsule. Potency ranges from 10 milligrams on the low end to 50 milligrams on the high end. Some people also like the flavor-free aspect compared to a typical tincture. Another plus: taking supplements or medication in capsule form is familiar to most people, unlike a daily ritual of placing drops of oil under your tongue.

What we might call CBD-plus capsules are a growing subset of this category. These products usually contain a moderate amount of CBD, such as 15 milligrams per capsule, and other ingredients that are said to complement the CBD. For example, capsules marketed as sleep aids might include melatonin, chamomile, and/or valerian. Another typical formulation is to add curcumin (turmeric), lion's mane mushroom, and other substances touted as natural anti-inflammatories to CBD. Perhaps inevitably, CBD is now also a primary ingredient in nootropics, the tech industry's go-to type of supplement for greater mental acuity. Products in this line combine CBD with plant extracts such as gingko balboa, water hyssop, and rosemary.

Because a capsule goes through the normal digestive process, it will probably take more than an hour for its CBD to enter your bloodstream. Time your consumption accordingly if you take capsules to help with sleep. Philip Blair, MD, a family physician in Vancouver, Washington, sometimes counsels his patients to chew on capsules in the hope of having the CBD metabolized more quickly.

Topical Solutions

Most CBD brands targeting active people offer one or more types of topical solutions, such as creams, lotions, salves, and serums. Companies with a broader health and wellness focus usually do as well, but these are more often things like lip balm or moisturizer. The key differences are that the sports topicals are designed to penetrate the outer layer of your skin, and their CBD concentration will be much higher than in their health and beauty counterparts.

Unlike CBD ingested orally, topicals are intended to deliver CBD to a specific body part or area. "Anecdotally, I have patients who swear by topical CBD application for underlying joint pain and tendinopathy," says Boston-based sports dermatologist Robin Travers, MD. The goal is to address site-specific inflammation rather than attempt to lower the body's overall inflammatory process.

Sports podiatrist Charlton Woodly, of Fort Worth, Texas, says, "It just makes sense that if I have pain in my Achilles tendon I would apply something to my Achilles tendon instead of taking something orally, especially when you are able to manipulate that cream on a muscle or joint, increasing blood flow and breaking up a little bit of scar tissue with light massage."

Apply topicals wherever you're having particular issues. I've noticed much more benefit when I consistently apply topicals two or three times a day—say, after showering and before going to bed—than once.

Let's step back a bit and consider a basic question: How do any topical solutions, whether or not they contain CBD, work?

There's no doubt that some topical applications can help with internal inflammation. Prescription-only patches and gels containing nonsteroidal anti-inflammatories are increasingly popular, given concerns about the effect of traditional anti-inflammatories on internal organs. Later in this chapter, we'll look at the matter of CBD's bioavailability— that is, how much of what you take ultimately winds up in your bloodstream. Topicals theoretically bypass this issue by not first going through your gastrointestinal system. So if CBD has anti-inflammatory properties, the right kind of topical should help with site-specific inflammation.

The first, obvious requirement of an effective topical solution is that the active ingredients penetrate the skin. "An oil or cream is likely to penetrate the skin better than a petroleum-based topical like Tiger Balm," says sports podiatrist Brian Fullem, of Clearwater, Florida. The overwhelming majority of CBD topicals marketed to athletes meet this criteria. Most include ingredients, such as beeswax or eucalyptus oil, that help the solution get through to deeper tissue levels, so that the CBD can enter the bloodstream and/or work directly on the targeted soft tissue, such as a tendon.

Next, consider the application site. How much gets absorbed varies by body part. "The skin can be considered a multilayered biological membrane, with specific absorption characteristics at various layers," says Travers. "Dry skin will have different absorption characteristics than well-hydrated skin. Thick calloused skin has a thick external layer that differs from smooth, thinner skin, such as on the face. Diseased skin (such as from eczema or psoriasis) will have different absorption abilities than intact skin."

Travers cites some research that has found greater bioavailability of CBD via topicals than oral solutions. "It remains unclear whether the improvements in underlying joint pain are by direct transfer of the CBD from the skin to the cannabinoid receptors in the underlying joint, or through systemic vascular absorption and delivery through the normal blood supply to the joint," she says.

There's a second big factor involved in any topical solution's effectiveness. As Fullem says, a popular product like Tiger Balm probably doesn't get past the surficial skin layers. Yet it certainly feels like something is happening, and many people swear by Tiger Balm, IcyHot, and similar topicals for short-term pain relief. What's going on?

"I think the placebo effect is very much in play with topicals," Scott Palmer, MD, a team physician for the Chicago White Sox and Chicago Bulls, says. "They can have fragrances and consistencies that makes you think, 'I think this is going to help.' Bengay, Tiger Balm, they're counterirritants. You get a warm, tingly feeling when you put it on a joint. It's probably doing nothing for the inflammation, but it's helping your brain make it like you're feeling better."

Justin Young, who develops products for Floyd's of Leadville, says, "Why do they have ingredients like lavender or mint? The aroma tells your brain that something different is going on. It distracts your mind from the pain. There's definitely a placebo effect going on."

Young isn't admitting that topicals don't "work" in the sense of lowering inflammation. It's pretty clear that, with the right formulation, CBD can penetrate deeply enough to work its anti-inflammatory magic. As we'll see in a bit, when Palmer, Young, and others talk about the placebo effect, they mean something different—and more positive— than most of us do.

Topicals are a great choice for athletes. For many of us, they're an add-on to regular oral CBD consumption, applied on an as-needed basis. (I will admit that after several consecutive days of slipping around on snowy runs in the Maine winter, it would sometimes be simpler to say where I'm not applying it.) For others, topicals are the only form of CBD they use. That can be so for a variety of reasons: these athletes want help with chronic sore spots but feel they don't need to take something to improve sleep and recovery or reduce anxiety; they don't like the idea of taking supplements, no matter how natural; and/or they're concerned about consuming trace amounts of THC.

Drink Powders

There's no better sign of CBD's journey from head shop to sports shop than the growing number of drink powders targeted to athletes.

There are two main sports-oriented types: traditional sports drink powders with CBD added and flavor-free powders that can be added to anything. Floyd's of Leadville was an early innovator in the first category, offering a recovery protein powder (in vanilla or chocolate) and a berry-flavored electrolyte powder. As with many sports drink powders, regardless of whether they contain CBD, these are best appreciated for their benefit rather than stand-alone taste.

The flavor-free options are so versatile they become more than just drink powders. I've added them not only to water, coffee, tea, smoothies, and kombucha but to oatmeal, cereal, yogurt, soup, and other foods. Think of these powders as good for busy, wellness-conscious people (which athletes obviously are) who will appreciate the portability and convenience. The same is true of flavored powders not specifically marketed as sports drinks. Citrus and cocoa are the main flavors here. The few that are full-spectrum have a slight cannabis taste, so of course my wife and I joke about having a nice soothing cup of "pot cocoa."

Powder potency varies, as with other product types. The Floyd's electrolyte powder supplies 5 milligrams of CBD per provided quarter-cup scoop, while the recovery protein powder contains 25 milligrams in the same size scoop. The flavor-free powder from another athlete-oriented company, Oleo, contains 25 milligrams of CBD in the provided half-teaspoon scoop. Various brands' individual serving packets meant to be mixed with 16 ounces of liquid typically contain 10 to 15 milligrams of CBD.

Other Edibles

At the other end of the spectrum from a CBD protein powder are edibles such as gummy bears. With all the ways to consume CBD, I don't think that buying a package of sugary gummy bears is a top go-to means for athletes. The same goes for chocolate bars with CBD, and that's without considering that a one-ounce bar can cost $10 to $20.

Some brands offer edible concentrates that go by descriptors like *crumble* or *shatter.* These come packaged as little flakes that you—wait for it—crumble or shatter into smoothies, drinks, and other foods. As concentrates, they're strong. A typical small jar, about the size of a lip balm container, will pack 750 to 1,000 milligrams of CBD into less than a teaspoon of flakes. Most have interesting flavors (cherry wine, gelato, pineapple, etc.) while still carrying a strong cannabis taste. They're an easy but expensive (about $50 per small jar) way to add CBD to your diet. Using the right amount can be tricky; because the products are so concentrated, they can overwhelm the taste of whatever you're adding them to.

I find it easier to satisfactorily integrate less concentrated products. I've had a honey with 400 milligrams of CBD added to a four-ounce jar. That works out to a little more than 15 milligrams of CBD per teaspoon. In this case the cannabis taste of the CBD gave the honey an extra, complementary layer of flavor. With the small jar costing $50, I had incentive to use it sparingly rather than take my usual by-the-spoonful-from-the-jar approach. I've also tried coconut oil with added CBD. It makes a nice addition to smoothies, baked goods, and other homemade foods. But the 12-ounce bottle contains 150 milligrams of CBD. To get any significant effect from consuming the coconut oil, you'd probably need to eat more of it at once than most of us are up for.

CBD added to single-serving "normal food"—cookies, brownies, et cetera—is a growing phenomenon in many urban areas. These aren't your best regular go-to choice for the purposes of this book. Not that I have anything against cookies, as my neighborhood bakery can attest. But as with gummy bears, leaning on sweets as your go-to CBD vessel probably won't advance your athletic career. There's also the matter of knowing how much CBD you're getting and its type and origins. The same goes for typical coffees, teas, smoothies, and the like with CBD added to them. You're most likely getting about five milligrams of CBD, which isn't going to do much for active-lifestyle purposes by the time it's digested. Better to buy the normal cookie, enjoy it for its own sake, and devote the extra two dollars you would have spent on the CBD cookie to buy your own CBD and take it on your terms.

Suppositories

Didn't see this one coming, did you?

Neither did I when I started working on this book. But here we are—some companies that sell the usual forms of CBD also offer rectal and vaginal suppositories. Suppositories are a go-to means of administering medications for people with local GI conditions, such as ulcerative colitis or Crohn's disease, or when taking medicine by mouth is impractical, as in cases of severe nausea or vomiting. But the claim is that overall, other than injections, suppositories are the most efficient way to get a desired product into the bloodstream.

I tried suppositories on several occasions. My first experience was on a holiday when I told myself I should be working (on this book!) but was looking for an excuse to do otherwise. About half an hour after administering the suppository, I felt a deep sense of calm and relaxation. My mind stopped its angel-devil discussion of whether I should be working. The overall feeling was akin to how you might feel after a massage or a soak in an Epsom-salt tank.

For my next experiment, I administered a suppository instead of ingesting my usual prebed oral CBD. My notes from the following morning read "great sleep!" and "got up later than usual." As always in these sorts of trials, it's impossible to know what would have been the case otherwise. But I've yet to have a bad night's sleep after using a suppository. In daytime, I use them only if I know not much is expected of me the next few hours. It's not that they're incapacitating; rather, to continue the massage parallel, I want to be able to enjoy and absorb the benefits of the restorative experience. But that's just me. I know a suppository aficionado who is, overall, a more anxious person than I am. She appreciates the calm clarity that suppositories bring when she's struggling to focus on important work.

As with so many things concerning CBD, I'm unaware of hard data showing that suppositories result in greater bioavailability than the same amount of CBD administered otherwise. Medical professionals I consulted differed on the topic. Erin Dawson-Chalat, MD, an ob-gyn in Portland, Maine, told me that, in general, suppositories deliver more of a given substance than oral consumption. On the other hand, Palmer said, "I don't buy the concept of increasing serum CBD concentrations via rectal delivery. The limited bioavailability of CBD is the same whether it's delivered to gastric or rectal mucosa."

The suppositories I tried contained either 50 milligrams or 100 milligrams; these are relatively high amounts to take at once. For comparison, if you have a standard one-ounce tincture that contains 300 milligrams of CBD, taking 100 milligrams at once would entail swallowing 10 droppers. So is it the means of delivery or the amount that's most at play here? That's unclear, but when I've taken 50 or 100 milligrams of CBD at once via tincture, capsule, or drink powder, I haven't felt as (pleasantly) affected as after the suppositories.

If (as I was) you're new to suppositories, the answer is no, it doesn't hurt.

Vaping and Everything Else

I know that some will disagree with me here, but of the most popular ways to take CBD, vaping seems the most antithetical to an athletic lifestyle. In addition to the smoke, there are the chemicals in the vaping liquid. Also, a study about CBD labeling that we'll look at in Chapter 3 found that vaping solutions were the most likely of various product types to be mislabeled. None of the athletes I interviewed for this book told me they regularly vape CBD. Of course, most of us do things that aren't ideal for the athletic part of our lives; there are about 17 things wrong with my posture as I type this sentence. But that doesn't make it okay to include those practices in an athlete-focused book. That's my story, and I'm sticking to it!

Even less pertinent to athletic use are the many standard home and bath products that can now be found with added CBD. I like pampering myself at least as much as the next person. But don't expect to be fresher for your next workout thanks to offerings such as bath bombs, candles, lip balms, moisturizers, shampoo, deodorant, toothpaste, conditioner, or eye balm.

Of course, you're not obligated to take CBD in just one form. Many of the athletes I spoke with for this book mix it up, usually with a regimen of tincture or capsule on a daily basis and topical applications as needed. Tim Drennan, who makes CBD products for several brands, including his own, MYKU Wellness, says, "If you're finding CBD isn't working for you, think about changing the method of application. If tinctures aren't bringing relief, try a lotion, or a gel cap. Everybody has their Goldilocks zone."

Product type can also vary by situation. I leave tinctures at home when travel involves flying. Although the standard bottles are well under the Transportation Safety Administration's 3.4-ounce limit for carry-ons, and even though the TSA page doesn't list hemp oil as a prohibited carry-on substance, the slight chance that a $70 tincture will get flagged during screening just isn't worth the risk for me. If I feel I want a supplementary dose after a particularly long or hard workout, I tend toward drink powders. I'm going to be downing a lot of fluid in the aftermath of a draining run anyway, so mixing some powder into a drink feels like a better route than taking one or two droppers of CBD oil.

For people who struggle to exercise consistently, the answer to the question "What's the best type of workout?" is usually "The one you're most likely to do." The same principle applies with taking CBD—start with the form that you're most likely to consume consistently enough to see if it helps.

How Much CBD to Take

An adage in my sport, running, says that we're all an experiment of one. That thought applies to how much CBD to take to get your desired effect. "One of the intricacies of CBD is that effective dosing can be much different between two people," Michael Lewis, MD, of Bethesda, Maryland, says. "There's no way to know what dose is right for you until you try it."

Here's another adage: start low and slow. That's the general medical advice for any new medication or supplement. For CBD, that means beginning on the low end of regular users' daily amounts, such as 5 to 15 milligrams. If you're using a tincture, that will be part or all of one dropper of a standard-potency oil. "If you're feeling no effects, adverse or beneficial, after three to five days, add another serving of the same amount," Lewis says.

Blair advises a similar gradual ramp-up. "If you respond to the initial dose, that's fine, you don't need to do more," he says. "If you don't get the relief you seek after a week or so, double the dose. If that's still ineffective after another week, double the dose again. If someone does that and they still feel no benefit, I'll say, 'I'm not sure it's going to be effective for you.'"

Lewis and others recommend starting with taking a dose in the hour before you go to bed. That makes sense, given that one common goal is improved sleep. Also, as we'll see in a bit, a sign that you're taking too much is lethargy or grogginess, and it's better to deal with that at the end of your day than when you need to be most productive.

There are two big caveats to the above advice on how much to take. First, says Lewis, there's great variance in how people respond to any substance. "Some people have a hyper metabolism," he says. "They're very sensitive to things going in their body or on their skin. Others can take a large dose of most medications and they might not feel much. There's no way to know with CBD until you try it, but if you're sensitive to most medications, start at the lower end of typical doses."

A second consideration is that athletes will probably wind up wanting to take more than the average sedentary person who isn't pushing herself hard day after day. Floyd's of Leadville owner Bob Bell says that the company's 50-milligram soft gels are its top seller. Clare O'Nan, an acupuncturist and naturopathic doctor in Starkville, Mississippi, says, "I don't usually recommend what's on the bottle because it's usually too little. For most athletic people, I advise starting with the minimum serving size and then dosing up quickly until they get to the highest level of effectiveness."

How much is too much? Hector Lopez, MD, says no significant adverse reactions have been reported for the more than one million doses that have been sold in the

United States. There is, however, a personal threshold at which the products stop being effective and maybe even become less effective. The most common sign that you're taking too much is fatigue. "If you're feeling tired and washed out, back off," Lewis says.

In my first weeks of taking CBD, I experimented with a wide range of doses. I found I was too sedate during work hours if, on a typical day, I took CBD in the morning and at night. A dose of 25 milligrams in the hour before going to bed, plus as-needed topical use, has become my norm. The main exception is after an especially long or hard weekend run, when I have an additional 25 milligrams if I'm planning to mostly lounge about the house.

Once you've found your milligrams-per-day sweet spot, will that change over time? After all, regular marijuana users are well aware of building tolerance and needing more to get the same effect. It's natural to wonder if the same thing happens with this nonintoxicating cannabinoid.

What little research there is on the topic suggests regular CBD use doesn't lead to tolerance. A Japanese study on mice found that, in these rodents as in humans, more THC was eventually needed to produce the desired benefit (in this case, protection from some of the consequences of reduced blood flow to the brain). The researchers found that repeated treatment with THC desensitized the mice's CB1 receptors. In contrast, they found, regular CBD intake didn't desensitize CB1 receptors, presumably because CBD did its work through other neural pathways.

A theoretical argument could even be made that, over time, you might need less CBD to get your desired benefits. The thinking here is that a few months of regular CBD intake increase your body's level of endocannabinoids, similar to some people's belief that a short-term diet heavy in lacto-fermented food can boost your gut's microbiome. Once reset, these systems might continue to operate at a higher level without as much external help (and as much toll on your wallet).

Some practitioners have incorporated this approach into their CBD recommendations. "I don't like to keep people on CBD if it's not absolutely necessary," says Ashley Mayer, a naturopathic doctor and World Masters Champion swimmer in Scottsdale, Arizona. "That's my philosophy with most medications—to slowly wean people off them." Similarly, O'Nan says, "I recommend that athletic people stay at their most effective level for three to four months and then try to back down."

A consideration here is why you're taking CBD. If it's to address a specific injury, a good amount for a few months might be enough to get you over the hump, after which time you could conceivably continue to thrive on a lower dose or none at all. On the other hand, if you're training ambitiously and perhaps are not as young as you used to be, and you feel CBD helps you do what you want to do, you might continue your current dosage for the foreseeable future. "A lot of the athletes I see feel chronic wear and tear, so they're always on it, and that's fine," Mayer says.

When to Take CBD

CBD has many potential uses, and its effects are generally more subtle than instantly noticed. So when to take it for maximum effectiveness isn't necessarily as important as is the case with something like an antihistamine.

Still, it doesn't hurt to experiment with taking CBD at different times of day, depending on what your reasons for using it are. Here are some rough guidelines on timing your dosage. We'll cover some of these scenarios in more detail in later chapters.

Why You're Taking CBD	When to Take It
Sleep	Half an hour to an hour before going to bed if using tincture; one to two hours before going to bed if using capsule
General anxiety	Half an hour to an hour before starting the busiest part of your day
Task-specific anxiety	Half an hour to an hour before an acutely stressful situation
General pain and inflammation	Any time of day, but consider starting with soon after working out
Acute pain and inflammation	Apply a topical solution after working out and two or three other times during the day
Overall recovery from training	Any time of day, but consider starting with soon after working out
Acute recovery from training	Integrate into food or drink within the first 30–90 minutes following your longest and/or hardest workouts

How Much CBD Are You Really Getting?

One challenge to finding your personally effective dosage is that CBD has low bioavailability. That is, there's a big difference between how many milligrams of CBD you consume and how much eventually makes its way into your bloodstream so that it can do its thing throughout your body.

"The oral bioavailability of CBD is actually quite low because it undergoes extensive first-pass metabolism," Travers says. "This means that, when it is absorbed through the gastrointestinal tract, it is metabolized heavily by the liver before it even gets a chance to get to the target organs."

Palmer says, "The CBD molecule is very, very lipophilic [literally, fat-loving], but it's sort of hydrophobic [water-hating]. It gets into fat really well, but it doesn't like the water environment. So it doesn't get very well absorbed from the GI tract, and once it does get absorbed the liver chews it up."

It's estimated that the bioavailability of a typical oral CBD product (tincture, capsule, etc.) is only about 8 to 10 percent. So if you take a dropper of CBD oil that contains 20 milligrams of CBD, only about 2 milligrams gets to your nerve receptors, pain receptors, central nervous system, and brain.

There are two main ways to try to increase CBD's bioavailability—how you take it, and how products are made. We saw above that some people believe suppositories result in more CBD reaching target areas. Topical solutions are also an attempt to bypass the gastrointestinal tract. Taking tinctures sublingually theoretically allows some absorption through mucous membranes in the mouth; the same goes for oral solutions administered as a spray.

In terms of product development, several companies are trying to find ways to get more CBD through the GI tract. These efforts generally involve encapsulating the CBD molecule and/or shrinking the size of the particles that make their way from your mouth to the rest of your body. It must be said that these companies often present the superiority of their delivery mechanism as a given, without much more evidence than the theoretical basis for their approach. In these early days of a mass CBD market, the best summation of the issue is that brands know low bioavailability is a potential barrier to product efficacy, and ones that can prove greater bioavailability will likely be rewarded with more customers.

For now, it's worth asking: If such low amounts of CBD are available from typical usage, is anything really happening? Before you dismiss claimed benefits as "just a placebo effect," consider what the placebo effect is.

In Praise of Placebos

Most people misunderstand the placebo effect. They'll say, "Oh, that's just a placebo effect" to mean that something—a medication, a form of treatment, a diet—doesn't cause improvements and is a waste of time. You might tell a friend you've been sleeping much better since starting to take CBD and be told to save your money because it's just a placebo effect.

That's not how it works. As touched on before, the gold

standard for research is a double-blind study with a control group. Half of the subjects receive the substance being researched, such as a medication. The other half (the control group) receive something that doesn't contain the substance but is otherwise identical, such as a pill that's the same size, color, and taste as the trial medication. *Double-blind* means that during the trial period neither the subjects nor the researchers know who's in the trial group and who's in the control group.

The point of a trial like this is to see whether the people in the trial group have better outcomes than those in the control group. For example, for a test of a cholesterol medication to be considered successful, cholesterol readings of those in the trial group should decrease significantly more than for those in the control group. Note the "significantly more" qualifier. In almost all studies with this design, some people in the control group realize a benefit, even though they've received what should be an inefficacious substance. That's the placebo effect.

In other words, the placebo effect measures real improvements. In some trials of Viagra, the erectile-dysfunction drug performed about 50 percent better than the placebo. That's a significant difference, but for our purposes here, the relevant outcome is that men taking a pill that had no conceivable mechanism to affect erectile dysfunction nonetheless saw improvement. Or consider antidepressants. Trials have repeatedly found those in the control group to report fewer depressive symptoms. Anecdotally, many of us have heard from friends who start taking an antidepressant and report feeling significantly better within a few days, even though modern antidepressants, which have a long half-life, should take a couple of weeks to really work on the targeted brain chemistry.

The placebo effect is thought to happen because of one's belief in the substance or treatment in question. It's a reminder of how integrated our physical and psychological well-being are. More than most people, athletes should be well aware of, and eager to capitalize on, the power that can come from the idea that you're doing something to improve your situation.

"I love the placebo effect," Fullem says. "I don't care if it's you or the treatment, as long as you're getting better." As a sports podiatrist, Fullem is a proponent of shockwave therapy for chronic foot and ankle tendon injuries. "When I start using it with a patient, I try to be positive. I'll say, 'It might not work right away, but I'm confident this will help you.' That affirmation can make a difference. I've had patients tell me after two weeks they're feeling better, even though the real effects of shockwave therapy should take about six weeks to kick in."

Palmer says of the placebo effect, "We embrace it, because if people feel better, that's the goal. If you feel that you're doing the right thing for yourself, that's mentally a good thing, and if you follow through with the physical improvements, then you've benefited."

Even if you've pooh-poohed the placebo effect, you've probably seen it in action in sports, and in your own regimen. Think about athletes who join a new team, or who start working with a different coach, and within a few weeks perform much better. Barring doping, it's doubtful that they massively increased their physical capacity in that short time. It was more likely that the change of narrative—I'm out of that old situation, this new one will be better—allows their latent potential to emerge. Similarly, you might have times where you might have reached a new level after a seemingly small change in your workout routine or diet.

Palmer's last point—"if you follow through with the physical improvements"—is also pertinent here. CBD might help to set the right process in motion. Then it's up to you to build on that confluence of belief and action that lies behind all breakthroughs. As I'll relate in more detail in Chapter 4, soon after I started taking CBD, the knee pain that had bothered me for a year began to improve. I was then able to regularly do strengthening exercises and other rehab to regain full function. This positive cycle fed on itself, including psychologically, as the more improvement I saw, the more motivated I was to keep working to get better.

As Fullem said when we discussed the placebo effect, if you feel better, you feel better. To a certain extent, who cares why?

Key Points on How to Take CBD

- Tinctures and capsules are the best choices for regular consumption by athletes.
- You'll need to experiment to find your optimal daily dose.
- More isn't necessarily better. Taking too much CBD can interfere with your workouts by making you groggy.
- Topical solutions are an excellent choice for athletes looking to treat site-specific pain and inflammation.

Chapter 3

How to (Smartly) Buy CBD

Let's say you're intrigued enough to try CBD. You've considered the various ways to take it and have a rough idea of how to start (when, how much, etc.). You go online to investigate your buying options and . . .

You're overwhelmed. Whether you're looking for tinctures or powders, capsules or creams, you'll find a seemingly infinite number of options. Prices, strength, and supposed benefits are all over the place. At the same time, your eyes can glaze over because so many products seem alike; which of the 73 one-ounce tinctures that your search suggested should you get?

You can also get incapacitated by too many choices in a store. That was my experience the first time I bought CBD. Not knowing any better, I asked for a tincture. I now realize that's akin to walking into Whole Foods and asking for a piece of organic produce. The salesperson showed me a dozen or so options while saying all sorts of things that meant nothing to me at the time. I went with the least expensive one (and now realize I got what I paid for).

Things don't have to be so confusing. Here's how to be a savvy CBD shopper.

Choose a Product Type (or Two)

As we saw in the previous chapter, CBD is making its way into an ever-growing range of products. But as we also saw, there are a handful that are most likely to be effective additions to your active lifestyle. So while bath bombs and lip balms might make nice Valentine's Day presents, let's focus on the types most pertinent to athletes.

If you're going to take CBD orally, your main choice is between tinctures and capsules. (See the previous chapter for why I'm omitting vape and food products here.) Tinctures are probably the better choice if you're new to CBD. You'll be able to experiment with different dosages more easily. Taking capsules will mean limiting yourself to whatever the amount per pill is. Put another way, tinctures are digital, capsules are analog.

Capsules might be a better choice if you have an idea how much CBD per day works for you. They're also preferable if swallowing a (usually) flavor-free pill is more appealing than placing an odorous oil under your tongue.

Some athletes are interested primarily in site-specific help with injuries or chronic sore spots. Topicals are the best starting point in these cases.

If you're convinced CBD works for you, a range of product types can be best. I find the combination of an oral (usually tincture) and topical to best address my goals of improved sleep, lowered overall inflammation, and TLC for acute problem spots.

Choose Full-Spectrum or Isolate

Almost all products will be described as "full-spectrum" or "isolate." This distinction doesn't have to do with how strong or concentrated a product is. The difference: full-spectrum products contain not only CBD but additional cannabinoids and other parts of the hemp plant, including terpenes (plant chemicals that impart flavor and fragrance) and flavonoids (plant chemicals that impart color). In isolate products, CBD is the only part of the hemp plant present. (There will be other ingredients, such as the coconut oil in tinctures that carries the CBD.)

Advocates of full-spectrum products tout the "entourage effect," which is another way to say that the various components of the plant work together to be more than the sum of their parts. For example, flavonoids in fruits and vegetables are widely believed to have antioxidant and anti-inflammatory properties; theoretically, these benefits should accrue in addition to whatever anti-inflammatory work CBD does.

Tim Drennan, who develops products for several CBD brands, including his own, MYKU Wellness, explains the entourage effect with an analogy. "Think of the receptors in your brain as light switches," he says. "Some combination of on, off, and neutral will get a blue light to appear. You take a CBD isolate, and it hits maybe 70 of 400 receptors, but the blue light doesn't come on. So you try a broad-spectrum product—CBD with a few other cannabinoids. Now maybe 200 of the 400 switches are being used, and you get a faint blue light. So you try a full-spectrum product. Now all 400 switches are being activated in some way, and you get the strong blue light you want."

On a theoretical level, the entourage effect makes sense, in the same way that you're better off eating an orange than taking a vitamin C pill—the orange will include fiber, juice, and other parts of the plant that evolved to coexist. At the same time, even someone like Drennan is wary of how the supposed advantage of full-spectrum products is stated as a fact.

"There's a lot of hippie science in the hemp industry," he says. "There's no peer-reviewed research right now that proves the entourage effect is better on something like inflammation. I have consumer metrics that show a positive trend toward broad- and full-spectrums being more efficacious than isolates. But there's not the hard science yet."

It's possible that hard science will never exist. In Chapter 1 we saw how nonuniformity among whole-plant-derived products makes replicable research difficult. "The FDA is never going to approve as medicine products that vary from batch to batch, that you can't quantify precisely," says Scott Palmer, MD. "It's convenient to say there's an entourage effect, but nobody can precisely define it because nobody's ever separated out all the isolates and then recombined them to show the best mix. Nobody does that because nobody has the time or money, so they just say it's the mixture of the components that works."

The primary concern with full-spectrum products is that THC, the cannabinoid responsible for a marijuana high, will likely be present in trace amounts. (Remember, by definition hemp contains no more than 0.3 percent THC.) In CBD products that contain what they claim—more on that in a bit—the amount of THC present isn't enough to give you a buzz. It's possible, however, that these trace amounts could trigger a false positive result for marijuana use if you're subject to workplace or other drug testing.

Unless you're concerned about potentially consuming trace amounts of THC, there's no real reason not to buy full-spectrum. (In some brands, isolate tinctures and capsules are about five dollars less expensive than the full-spectrum version of the same potency.) The main exception in this regard are powders, which will usually be CBD isolates. These are likely to be the sort of thing you branch out into once you've established whether CBD works for you.

Consider the Manufacturing Process

The most common method used to get CBD and other cannabinoids from a hemp plant into something you buy is called supercritical CO_2 extraction. Pressurized carbon dioxide pulls out the plant's desired contents, with the caveat that the extraction process isn't 100 percent effective. (Talk to industry insiders, and they'll bemoan the loss of some terpenes and flavonoids during extraction.) This method is the current industry standard because it's relatively efficient and doesn't involve using a solvent, resulting in the basis for an all-natural product.

Some companies use different processes with the goal of increasing bioavailability. Remember from the previous chapter that it's widely believed that about only 10 percent of the CBD you take in oral form enters your bloodstream. The CBD molecule is "hydrophobic," meaning that it tries to move away from water, but "lipophilic," meaning that it's soluble in fat. These alternative methods trap CBD molecules in a colloidal solution that, theoretically, allows for better transport through the body. Look for words like "liposome" or "lipid-infused."

Another alternative is to trap the CBD molecule in a water-soluble shell. For example, Oleo, which offers CBD isolate in powder form, calls its process "micro-encapsulation." Oleo's site provides the results of a mechanical model that shows greater absorption of their product. It's reasonable to think that would also happen in humans, but so far this is unproven.

The nexus of the manufacturing process and bioavailability can be tricky to navigate. "The broad range of available formulations on the market make the degree of specific improvement unknown," says Palmer. The onus is on companies to prove that their processes lead to greater CBD absorption in humans. Until that proof exists, claimed differences in bioavailability on the basis of manufacturing processes aren't something to get too hung up on.

Calculate Your Desired Dose

Knowing how much CBD you're taking can involve a little math. Again, capsules are straightforward—the package will usually say how much CBD each one contains. Occasionally, the (slightly irritating) presentation will be total amount of CBD and number of capsules, such as 450 milligrams and 30 capsules, in which case it's up to you to do the quick calculation that each capsule contains 15 milligrams.

For tinctures, you need to know the total amount of CBD in the container and the container's size to calculate how much CBD is in each serving. A typical tincture bottle contains 30 milliliters (roughly one ounce) of CBD oil. A typical serving is one dropper, or 0.3 milliliters, meaning that each such bottle contains 30 servings. So a tincture of this size that contains 300 milligrams of CBD will deliver 10 milligrams per dropper, a 600-milligram bottle will deliver 20 milligrams per dropper, and so on.

You can find tinctures of this size that contain 100 milligrams of CBD, ones that contain 3,000 milligrams of CBD, and everything between. That's quite a range! Most have between 300 and 600 milligrams. This information is crucial, because buying CBD isn't like perusing a selection of wines with varying alcohol content. With CBD, the potency is often the primary bit of data you're looking for.

Over the past year, more brands have started to offer higher-potency tinctures for people who have settled on a relatively high regular. These ultra-strength products make taking your desired amount of CBD more efficient, without swallowing several droppers of MCT coconut oil a day.

These calculations are much more difficult with topical solutions. Like tinctures, topicals vary greatly in potency. Unlike tinctures, they tend to also vary greatly in volume. One brand's salve contains 1,000 milligrams of CBD in 2.2 ounces. Another's cream has 700 milligrams in a 30-gram (1.05-ounce) container. Without doing the precise math, you can still see that these two products deliver higher amounts of CBD than another brand's balm (100 milligrams in 1.3 ounces) and a different company's cream (750 milligrams in 3.4 ounces).

But what makes buying topicals especially tricky is that it's harder to know what a typical "serving" is. Are you rubbing just a dab on one Achilles tendon, or slathering a large dollop on your right knee and left shoulder? Out of curiosity, I emptied one brand's two-ounce jar of cream. It contained roughly eight teaspoons; one teaspoon yielded enough cream for three solid swipes of my index finger. So this jar might last you a month, or you might go through it in a week.

Adding to the lack of precision with topicals are differences in consistency—you're likely to apply more of one that feels like whipped cream than a balm, and you'll probably put on even less of one that's more like a serum. And as we saw in the previous chapter, it's likely that a topical's other ingredients will affect how much CBD penetrates your skin. Given all these variables, it's probably best to buy topicals toward the stronger end of what's available. After all, if you're using one you probably have one or more specific spots in mind that need above-and-beyond attention.

Of course, all of this math is impossible if you don't know how much CBD is said to be in a package. And yet it's easy to find CBD products that don't say how many milligrams of CBD they contain. Would you buy sunscreen with an unknown SPF? Or a vitamin D pill that didn't state its strength in terms of International Units? As we'll see in a bit, knowing how much CBD is in any product can be tricky enough. Avoid any product that doesn't clearly state on its label either how much total CBD it contains (typical for tinctures and topicals) or how much CBD individual products contain (as with capsules).

Check the Ingredients

Any CBD product worth your money will list its ingredients on the package. This listing should be as clear as possible and should not require a degree in organic chemistry to decipher. Be wary of ingredient mumbo jumbo, such as "aqua" instead of "water" or "cera alba" in place of "beeswax." Such products might still be high quality, but you have to wonder why they're not being as transparent as possible. (Tangential remark from your middle-aged author: On the whole, CBD packaging has ridiculously small type, probably owing to trying to cram a lot of words onto tiny labels. You'll want to have your reading glasses handy if you're looking at labels in person.)

One site, the CBD Marketplace (cbdmp.com), has developed a list of criteria for the products it carries. The site advises buying only CBD products with all-natural ingredients and avoiding those that have artificial flavors, preservatives, parabens, dyes, vegetable glycerin, or propylene glycol. CBD Marketplace also recommends only CBD products that are sourced according to organic and non-GMO standards. These criteria are a good filter for any product, CBD or otherwise, that might help your health and athletic pursuits.

Consider the Claims

As we saw in Chapter 1, the federal Food and Drug Administration is closely monitoring the CBD industry. As of this writing, the FDA says that CBD doesn't meet the criteria for a dietary supplement; the reason is that CBD is an active ingredient in FDA-approved drugs and was researched in that vein before it was marketed as a dietary supplement. Nonetheless, it's easy to find the words "dietary supplement" on CBD product labels.

The FDA has sent warning letters to companies that claim unambiguous medical benefits for CBD, an especially egregious example being "cures cancer." Any product making those claims is, in the FDA's view, a drug for human use that has to go through the FDA approval process before it's marketed in the United States. Most CBD products' packaging now includes a disclaimer along these lines: "These statements have not been evaluated by the FDA. This product is not intended to diagnose, treat, cure, or prevent any disease."

Nonetheless, some companies claim that their products directly impart specific benefits. The packaging for one full-spectrum, 600-milligram tincture I tested read:

- Relieves pain and inflammation
- Supports brain function
- Reduces anxiety
- Improves sleep
- Relieves nausea

Contrast that with the promotional wording for another company's full-spectrum, 600-milligram tincture marketed to athletes:

- Takes the edge off the pain
- Helps you come back stronger

Similarly, another full-spectrum, medium-strength tincture I tried promises:

- May help relax the central nervous system and promote sleep
- May help the mind and body unwind

The three products are probably quite similar. Although in line with the letter of FDA guidelines, the first example above feels like a violation of the spirit of those guidelines. My athlete's hard-won skepticism—there are no magic bullets—inclines me toward trusting the second and third companies more. It's worth poking around a brand's site and packaging to see where its presentation of CBD lies on the spectrum of intellectual honesty. You'll be spending a fair amount of money; find brands whose ethos aligns with yours.

Double-Check the Ingredients

So you've gone to the trouble of figuring out what you want, at what strength, and you've found a product that has acceptable ingredients clearly stated on its label and that's free of overreaching claims. All set, right?

Unfortunately, no.

Consider an investigation into the topic published in the *Journal of the American Medical Association* in 2017. Researchers at the University of Pennsylvania Perelman School of Medicine purchased 84 CBD products made by 31 companies. They then removed the labels and sent the products to a lab to have the products' CDB and THC levels analyzed.

The results didn't inspire confidence. The researchers considered a product accurately labeled if its CBD content was within 10 percent of the claimed amount. Only 31 percent were. Close to half—43 percent—of the products were more than 10 percent short of the purported amount of CBD. (For example, a tincture said to contain 500 milligrams of CBD had less than 450 milligrams.) On the plus side, 26 percent of the products were at least 10 percent stronger than stated on the label.

Given the cost of most products, few of us will carp about getting more CBD than we think we're buying. THC, however, is another matter. The cannabinoid that triggers a marijuana high was detected in 18 of the 84 products tested. Remember, by definition, hemp contains no more than 0.3 percent THC; full-spectrum CBD products carry the slight chance that they'll contain a trace amount of THC. But some of the products, most likely because of sloppy sourcing, went beyond trace (in one case, 6.43 milligrams per milliliter). They were possibly strong enough "to produce intoxication or impairment, especially among children," the researchers wrote. That amount of THC could also theoretically show up if you're subject to workplace drug testing.

The solution: buy only products that have undergone third-party testing of the sort conducted in the University of Pennsylvania study. The results of these tests should be easy to find on a brand's website. Some products have a QR code on their packaging that leads to that batch's test results.

First, look to see that the amount of CBD claimed to be in the product is at least what the test shows. Depending on the product, this figure will either be for the total amount of CBD in a container, as with a tincture, or per item, as with a capsule. Then, if THC is a concern for you, look for that line on the results. You should see a value for "weight %." For products made with hemp, this figure shouldn't be greater than 0.3 percent.

Finally, some tests will show the results for heavy metals (arsenic, mercury, lead, etc.). Hemp plants soak up the constituents, good and bad, of the soil in which they're grown. That trait is why so many high-quality CBD brands use hemp grown on farms that use earth-friendly, if not organic practices. What you want to see on the test results is the word *pass* for the concentration of each metal tested. Of course, it's highly unlikely that a brand would post the results of a failed test and go ahead and sell that batch of CBD. So consider the heavy-metal test another sign of a brand's commitment to quality.

Consumers who demand this sort of transparency help the CBD industry weed out bad brands. The head of product development for one athlete-focused company told me it consistently aims to come in 5 percent over the stated amount, such as 630 milligrams in a tincture advertised as 600 milligrams, in part because they want good lab results to share with customers.

If you really want to go down a rabbit hole, you could look into the reputations of the companies doing the testing. But for most of us, it's reasonable to place more faith in a CBD company that freely offers lab results than one that doesn't. Further guidance should come later in 2019 when *Consumer Reports* publishes the results of its independent testing of several CBD products.

What You'll Spend

For products that meet the above criteria, here's a rough range of costs.

Tinctures (roughly one-ounce bottle)

- Low potency (100–300 milligrams of CBD per bottle): $25–$50
- Medium potency (500–600 milligrams of CBD per bottle): $50–$90
- High potency (900 or more milligrams of CBD per bottle): $85–$200

Capsules (30 per bottle)

- Low potency (10–15 milligrams of CBD per capsule): $40–$60
- Medium potency (20–25 milligrams of CBD per capsule): $45–$75
- High potency (50 milligrams of CBD per capsule): $90–$110

Because topicals vary so much in package size, it's harder to make direct comparisons. In general, expect to spend between $50 and $90 for a one- to three-ounce container, and expect the container to contain between 300 and 1,200 milligrams of CBD. Given the intended use of these products, the athlete's more-is-better mindset is probably a good guide here.

Some companies have started to offer tinctures in larger

containers. This move makes sense, given the increasing number of people who use CBD daily. Still, the industry standard for tinctures remains a roughly one-ounce bottle. Capsules and topicals also come primarily in smaller volume. People I spoke with at some brands confirmed that packaging size stems in part from concerns about sticker shock—$60 once a month for three months can feel like less of a financial hit than paying $180 all at once for a three-month supply. (Imagine a scenario where you bought all of your coffee for three months at once.)

In the final chapter, we'll see why and by how much experts think prices will come down in the next few years. For now, most people buying CBD have disposable income. There's no getting around that it seems expensive. On the other hand, if you feel real benefits, such that you perform better and enjoy your athletic pursuits more, well, how do you put a value on that?

Where to Buy

Most of us will start our tenure as CBD consumers online. That's a wise choice, given the opportunity to thoroughly investigate a brand's offerings and see if it appears reputable (based on matters such as sharing third-party testing and describing products in clear, hype-free language).

Once you're a regular CBD user, you'll probably still buy most products online, for the usual reasons of greater selection and convenience. This is not to downplay the benefits of in-person shopping. A good CBD retailer will let you sample products, which is appreciated given the cost.

You might also luck into finding a knowledgeable salesperson who can help fine-tune your CBD regimen.

For a quick checklist to refer to when shopping, see the Purchasing Checklist at the back of this book. Once you have your CBD in hand, it's time to see if it can help your active lifestyle. That's what we'll cover in the next four chapters.

Key Points on How to Buy CBD

- Start by picking one or two product types you're most likely to use regularly.
- Buy only products that state all ingredients in clear language on the label.
- Buy only products that have proof from third-party testing that they contain the claimed amount of CBD.
- Consider buying isolate rather than full-spectrum products if you are subject to drug testing or otherwise want to make absolutely sure you don't consume THC.

Chapter 4

CBD and Athletic Injuries

One of CBD's most-touted benefits is pain relief. In a survey of more than 2,000 Americans who take CBD, published in *Cannabis and Cannabinoid Research,* 62 percent said they used it to treat a medical condition; the top two conditions cited were "chronic pain" and "arthritis/joint pain."

Although the participants of this survey weren't exclusively athletes, the marketing of CBD increasingly emphasizes its potential as an active person's alternative to traditional pain relievers. Athletes, who can be a skeptical lot, are understandably leery of the dangers of both prescription pain medications and over-the-counter offerings.

We athletes also tend to be autonomous and are used to taking matters into our own hands. If something might help our workouts, we'll look into it. As mentioned in Chapter 1, a survey of CBD users found that only 10 percent learned about CBD from medical professionals. That finding meshes with how the CBD-for-pain message is spreading among active people—not from on high, but from athlete to athlete. In this chapter, we'll look at how CBD can help with the aches, pains, and injuries that come with regular exercise.

The Problem with Pain Meds

America's opioid problem is well documented and is rightly described as a crisis. Credible estimates put the number of Americans with an opioid disorder between two and four million, and the number of annual deaths by prescription medication overdose at around 15,000.

These stats might seem far removed from the athletic world most of us live in. But some key players in the CBD-for-athletes market have seen the problem up close.

Riley Cote played for the Philadelphia Flyers, a National Hockey League team, from 2006 to 2010. Since retiring, Cote has become an advocate of hemp for athletes. In addition to starting a CBD brand, BodyChek Wellness, he founded a nonprofit, Athletes for CARE, that helps professional athletes transition healthfully to the postretirement phase of their lives. A big issue for these former athletes, Cote says, is medical professionals' usual approach to pain management.

"The traditional protocol is a pill for this, a pill for that—opioids, sleep medicine, muscle relaxants," he says. "The exit strategy is then usually surgery, and more pills, and maybe dependency or addiction, and, if so, then into a treatment program. It's a dark cycle I've seen too often. BodyChek Wellness and Athletes for CARE is about a different approach, one that's preventative rather than rehabilitative, built around using CBD to manage pain, inflammation, anxiety, and sleep. I wanted to be on the right side of history and promote the solution."

Cote himself didn't become dependent on prescription pain medication. He used cannabis while playing and now uses it to manage the many injuries and chronic pain that came from being an enforcer on the ice. But he could well be talking about another retired pro athlete, Floyd Landis, in the above cautionary tale.

Landis, of course, was a cyclist who was stripped of his 2006 Tour de France title and banned from the sport for doping. While competing, Landis suffered a major hip injury in a crash. He had surgery for the injury in season and started taking opioids to manage the pain. Once banned, Landis had hip replacement surgery. The operation, other chronic pain, and severe depression over what had come of his life contributed to Landis becoming addicted to opioids. He credits cannabis with helping him overcome that addiction. Landis became such a believer in CBD's pain management power that he started the CBD company Floyd's of Leadville.

These are admittedly extreme examples. It's probable, however, that like me, you know someone who has "treated" decades-long pain with several ibuprofens a day.

Over-the-counter pain medicine might seem low risk, but the Food and Drug Administration has issued warnings about long-term use increasing the risk of heart attack and stroke. This class of medicine, known as nonsteroidal anti-inflammatory drugs, is also associated with increased risk of internal bleeding. "A lot of the traditional options have pretty bad long-term, and in some cases short-term, side effects, especially when it comes to the liver and kidney," says Charlton Woodly, a sports medicine podiatrist in Fort Worth, Texas. "Athletes rely on the kidneys a lot more than the average person."

That CBD might remove the need for traditional pain relievers is what initially attracted Andrew Talansky, a former Tour de France cyclist turned professional Ironman triathlete. "I don't like ibuprofen, I don't like prescription meds," he says. "I've always looked for natural alternatives."

Talansky was introduced to CBD in 2017 by cycling friends. "I didn't know anything about it, but I try to be open-minded," he says. As Talansky heard more testimonials from trusted sources, "[He] went from skeptical to intrigued to asking for advice." He started taking a capsule or tincture daily and applying a topical cream one to five times a day. "Within a week I noticed improvements in my chronic problem areas from using the topical cream," he says. "Now that I've been taking CBD for a while, I don't have weeklong flare-ups from my old cycling injuries."

Woodly says the medical profession might be on a similar skeptic-to-advocate trajectory. "CBD isn't yet something that I hear about a lot at professional conferences, but it's picking up steam," he says. "I believe primary care sports medicine physicians are especially starting to look into it because they and their patients are looking for alternatives to narcotics and other pain medications."

Another data point about CBD's unconventional route to the mainstream: Woodly incorporated topical CBD solutions into his practice after personal success. A former college athlete who now does jujitsu and teaches wrestling, Woodly is subject to shoulder, hip, and back pain. "I was looking for nonpharmacological ways to address all my bumps and bruises," he says. "A friend recommended it to me, I did some research, and decided to move forward. I saw enough benefit for myself that I added it to my practice."

Woodly says doctors might also have logistical motivation to be open to new, natural pain treatments. "We're seeing more and more regulation around prescription pain medications," he says. "There's more scrutiny and you have to jump through more hurdles to prescribe these medications, and probably rightfully so."

How CBD Might Help with Athletic Injuries

Into this growing disenchantment steps CBD. The promise of overcoming injuries and lowering pain and inflammation with no significant side effects sounds too good to be true. Is there any basis for this claim?

Published research on treating pain and inflammation in humans with CBD only (as opposed to CBD combined with THC, or THC only) is scant. The few human studies that have been done have focused on matters that researchers consider more important than, say, whether CBD can make your Achilles tendon feel good enough to try a trail run tomorrow. For example, a small study found that an oral CBD spray reduced reported pain levels in people with neuropathic pain from chemotherapy. Research on inflammation in humans has also focused on medical conditions, such as a study suggesting a promising role for CBD in people with inflammatory bowel disease.

The more pertinent research for our purposes here has been done on rodents. In general, the findings of animal studies should be seen as suggestive, not conclusive. We can't assume that rats acquire and experience inflammation and pain exactly as humans do. (For that matter, we can't assume that you and I feel pain similarly.) On the other hand, the placebo effect is not a factor in animal studies. If there are suggestions of less pain and inflammation, those findings are entirely due to physiological factors.

Here's a great example of a study in this area: University of Kentucky researchers used a standard laboratory means of inducing arthritis of the knee in rats. (Poor rats!) Then the researchers applied a topical CBD gel to the rats' knees for four days. The gel significantly reduced signs of inflammation, including joint swelling, immune cell response in the affected area, and the thickness of the synovial membrane (connective tissue lining the inner surface of the knee). The rats also appeared to be in less pain after treatment with the CBD gel. Their scores on a test of "paw withdrawal latency" (i.e., how sensitive they were to a pain stimulus) returned to almost prearthritis levels.

These and other findings, in human and animal studies, suggest that CBD can act systemically and locally to lower inflammation and pain. It's widely believed that CBD achieves these effects through the CB1 and CB2 receptors we covered in Chapter 1.

Dr. Palmer cites another route for CBD's effectiveness in relation to injuries—working similarly to the most popular non-narcotic pain medications.

When injury occurs, your body's immune system reacts by releasing chemicals that try to return the cells of the affected area to normal. The release of these chemicals leads to inflammation, which is marked by swelling, pain, heat, and redness. These signs of inflammation can be glaringly obvious, such as after an acute injury like a sprained ankle, or more subtle, such as during the more insidious onset of an overuse injury like Achilles tendinitis.

The enzymes that produce prostaglandins, a key part of the inflammatory response, are called cyclooxygenase, or COX. These enzymes are classified as COX-1 and COX-2. Standard pain medications are called COX inhibitors; they reduce inflammation and pain by inhibiting the production of prostaglandins. Ibuprofen and naproxen work on COX-1 and COX-2. Their nonselective action can be problematic. COX-1–produced prostaglandins protect the stomach and intestinal lining, so inhibition of them can lead to internal bleeding. Newer pain medications, such as Celebrex, are COX-2 inhibitors only.

"As it turns out, CBD is a very potent inhibitor of COX-1 and COX-2," Palmer says. "It appears to do this through a different pathway than typical pain drugs but to be quite effective at inhibiting those receptors, without the side effects." A review of the topic published in the journal *Pain and Therapy* adds that CBD has been shown to work directly on other key cell-surface receptors that are associated with pain and inflammation.

With the federal legalization of hemp and surging interest in CBD, there should be a lot more human research in this area in the near future. But as touched on in Chapter 1, it's likely to remain focused on medical conditions rather than athletic injuries. Studies in process before this book was published included CBD's effects on osteoarthritis of the hand, neuropathic pain in people with HIV, and ulcerative colitis. To get insight on using CBD for athletic injuries, we'll turn to sports medicine professionals who have incorporated it into their practices.

CBD and Specific Athletic Injuries

"I think of CBD being effective wherever inflammation is involved, whether that's the brain or the gut or the joints," says Hector Lopez, MD. "For athletes, that's where I'm most excited about CBD's potential—keeping inflammation under control."

Philip Blair, MD, also spoke broadly when I asked what sports injuries CBD might be most effective on. "You're being really specific in asking about joints and ligaments versus muscular injuries," he said. "I'm looking at it as impingement, where you're getting an inflammatory response. CBD can relieve that and improve functionality, and allow people to sleep at night, which is going to speed recovery."

Podiatrist Charlton Woodly was more specific, citing CBD's effectiveness at treating Achilles tendinitis and plantar fasciitis. (He uses only topicals, personally and professionally.) Charles Bush-Joseph, MD, a professor of orthopedics at Rush University Medical Center in Chicago, says, "I have found that patients receive benefit from topical use of CBDs with overuse tendon injuries of shoulders, knees, and ankles. While specific research on the use of CBD in this instance is lacking, many believe that it helps prevent muscle and collagen breakdown." The general consensus: CBD might be most effective in relieving site-specific inflammation and pain associated with standard overuse injuries, while also potentially lowering overall inflammation.

For those in contact sports, Blair says, "CBD might be able to prevent a lot of long-term problems from brain injuries. I put concussions in that category of mini-traumatic brain injury, because some of the same mechanisms are involved. CBD could stabilize that condition and advance recovery from those injuries."

Even more speculatively but equally intriguing, Lopez says CBD might have promise in healing bone injuries: both ones suffered acutely, like a broken collarbone from a bike crash, and stress fractures, which develop over time.

"There's preliminary data from rodent studies that CBD can improve bone remodeling after injury," he says. "The mechanism hasn't been elucidated completely, but the hypothesis is that the endocannabinoid system plays a role in the balance of osteoclasts [cells that break down old bone] and osteoblasts [cells that build new bone] responsible for healthy bone metabolism."

What typical sports injuries might CBD be less effective in addressing? Bush-Joseph says he's seen no benefit in patients with acute injuries such as muscle and ligament tears. From his realm, Woodly cites severe sprains, saying, "Nobody's rubbing anything on a person in that situation." Ashley Mayer, a naturopathic doctor in Scottsdale, Arizona, who works with a lot of athletes, says she hasn't seen an effect on runners and triathletes once they develop delayed-onset muscle soreness. (Whether CBD can help lessen the chance of developing delayed-onset muscle soreness is for Chapter 6.)

The idea of CBD being less effective on sudden sports injuries meshes with my experience. A few months after CBD seemed to provide significant relief to a months-long knee problem (more on that below), I wrenched my lower back while lifting weights. Running was impossible; even walking was problematic for a few weeks. I increased my CBD intake and regularly massaged my back and surrounding muscles with CDB topicals, to no avail. Only after taking prescription muscle relaxants could I resume my normal activities.

A Small Sampling of Athletes' Success with CBD

In interviewing a wide range of athletes for the book, I repeatedly heard about how they use CBD to manage their sport's aches and pains. I thought it would be valuable to share some of those stories to complement what we saw above about research and best practices:

Carol Pope is a lifelong endurance athlete who has done several Ironman triathlons and marathons and has completed the Race Across America bike race four times. The San Antonio, Texas, resident first heard about CBD in 2016 in, of all places, an *InStyle* magazine article. It described how celebrities applied CBD to the balls of their feet to be able to wear heels longer.

Pope bought a CBD topical solution immediately, not to increase her time in heels, but to treat chronic low-back pain from high mileage on the bike. "I noticed that it helped me—a lot," she says. Pope was surprised at the amount of relief CBD seemed to provide. She became sold on the overall idea of incorporating CBD into her regimen and started taking a medium-potency solution orally (in both oil and spray form) in addition to using a topical.

CBD hasn't inoculated Pope against injury. Now in her mid-50s, she sustained a meniscus tear during an Ironman training buildup. What CBD did for her, Pope says, was manage the injury. "I would experience significant pain when my miles increased," she says. "CBD helped get me through my workouts."

Pope plans to keep taking CBD for the foreseeable

future. Her meniscus tear hasn't healed, but it isn't an impediment to chasing her athletic goals, and she doesn't plan to have surgery. A bonus about her prebed CBD routine: "It helps me sleep," she says.

Chase Knight is the head trainer at Fitness Isn't Free, a CrossFit facility in Kansas City, Missouri. He heard competitors talking about CBD at the CrossFit Games in the summer of 2018. At the time, he associated CBD with marijuana. "Coming from a law enforcement family, I never smoked weed or did edibles," he says. "So my first thought about CBD was 'I don't need that stuff.' "

He changed his mind when Resilience, a CBD-for-athletes brand founded by military veterans, contacted him about carrying the brand at his gym. Knight had been in the army for a decade, and it was while he was stationed in Afghanistan that he became a CrossFit coach. "When I told my wife I was looking more into CBD," he says, "it turned out she'd been taking it for two months! She's a little more hippie/natural health than I am."

Knight trains one to two hours a day, depending on how busy his gym is. (CrossFit instructors run classes instead of participating in them.) He broke his back and injured his knee while in the military, and he has had surgery on both shoulders. So once he overcame his CBD-equals-marijuana concerns, he was eager to see if CBD could help his many chronic pain issues.

"I started taking one dropper [of a tincture] morning and evening and putting the CBD cream on anything that was sore, which for me can be a lot," he says. "At first I wasn't noticing much. But when I started using the cream two or three times a day, I started noticing a real difference in my aches and pains. Using it consistently is key for me.

My knees are never going to be 100 percent, but with the dropper morning and evening and the cream as needed, I get a fair amount of relief."

Nico Erickson-Deriso is a good example of an everyday athlete who finds CBD useful in addressing everyday aches and pains. A resident of New York City in his mid-20s, Erickson-Deriso was a sprinter in college and then transitioned to road races after graduation. He usually runs about 30 miles a week, more when he's training for longer races.

Erickson-Deriso uses only topical CBD. "I most often use it on my thighs and calf muscles after either an interval workout, a hill workout, or a long run—basically any time when I know that my legs are going to be a little bit achy the next morning," he says. "I have also found it to be especially effective in calming down my shin splints postworkout."

In line with the idea that CBD isn't a cure-all for athletic injuries, Erickson-Deriso says the topical he uses doesn't help much with masking strong, sharp pain. "The primary example I can point to here would be in relation to an acute groin strain I suffered," he says. "While the topical balm helped some when I was not moving, it failed to do much to mask the sharp pains I would feel when I would go up or down the stairs."

Kassia Meador has been a competitive surfer since age 15. In 2011, when she was 29, the Los Angeles resident placed second in the Association of Surfing Professionals women's longboard tour. (The Association of Surfing Professionals changed its name to the World Surf League in 2015.)

Meador first heard about CBD in its first big wave of attention, after the passage of the 2014 farm bill. She was intrigued by the many proposed benefits, including anti-inflammatory properties and pain relief. "I'm the type of person who always want to try things out for myself and have an opportunity to experience how my body reacts to and is supported by medicinal substances," she says.

Competitive surfing most definitely counts as a contact sport, with the contact occurring with the water and the board. In her first month of taking CBD, Meador found that her longtime shoulder, neck, and knee pain almost disappeared. She says that new injuries seem to heal faster since she had made a prebed tincture and as-needed topical use part of her training. "I have also received a lot of concussions from surfing, and CBD has helped significantly with cognitive function and postconcussion syndrome," Meador says.

Finally, me: My initial interest in CBD stemmed from wanting better sleep. That proposed benefit seemed plausible. I viewed the sports injury-specific claims with much more skepticism. Through my four decades of running and quarter century of writing about running, I've developed a reflective scoff toward quick fixes and miracle cures. Most running injuries are overuse injuries that develop over time and that often take at least as long to overcome.

When I started taking CBD, I'd been dealing for almost a year with the first knee injury of my running career. What started as vague stiffness and tenderness around the outside of my right knee eventually led to me being unable to run. An MRI showed that I had torn my lateral meniscus. After some more missed time, I was able to resume running but was still always conscious of the knee. A physical therapist gave me a series of exercises to do with the goal of shifting some of the load of running off the lateral meniscus. This was the spring of 2018. My plan was to have surgery in late 2018 if this conservative approach didn't work. By that summer I started mentally preparing myself for the operation.

Then I started taking CBD. My goal of improved sleep happened almost immediately. But soon after, I started noticing something else—my knee was no longer as creaky and tender. I could more comfortably move through a full range of motion. I wasn't constantly thinking about my knee every time I got up from sitting or took a tricky step. I could do the physical therapy exercises with no complaints from the knee, and I could add more ambitious strengthening work. About six weeks after starting to take CBD, I told my wife I was putting surgery on indefinite hold.

It's not that CBD "fixed" my meniscus tear. It's still torn. What CBD appeared to do was reduce inflammation at the site enough that the physical therapy work I was doing could take hold. I almost never think about the knee now; the primary exception is when I do squats or child's pose or some other activity that had been not just painful but impossible before. Then I think, "Hey, I'm doing what I want to do!"

How to Maximize CBD's Effectiveness in Treating Athletic Injuries

CBD can be part of your plan to minimize injuries' interference with doing your thing. But it's not a replacement for following sound injury prevention principles. Here are some general tips on avoiding and managing athletic injuries.

Be smart in the short term:
Stop your workout if you have a sudden soft tissue or bone pain that lasts more than a few seconds. (We all get those out-of-nowhere, gone-almost-immediately twinges from

time to time.) But a new pain that persists is a warning message.

If you have a lingering ache or limitation that makes it impossible to exercise without altering your usual technique, you need to address it. Continuing will not only worsen that issue but likely set off a cascade of compensatory woes elsewhere.

Be smart in the long term:

Determine why you developed an injury, and fix the underlying issue so that the injury doesn't recur.

Many of us are diligent about strengthening and stretching when we're coming back from injury. Then we tend to slack off on that work once we're back to doing what we love. And then we tend to get injured again. Commit to doing supplementary exercises a few times a week. Better to spend a little time in prehab than a lot of time in rehab.

Work on your overall athleticism:

Normal American adult life affords few opportunities to regularly move through a wide range of motion, as was the case during childhood. Most of us become adept at doing only the sport or sports we love, and increasingly constricted in other movements. Sitting several hours a day doesn't help. All of these factors increase our risk for injury. A good overall strength and flexibility program will build your overall athleticism. Trying new sports from time to time will also help, and you might even find other workouts you want to do regularly.

Watch your weight:

This doesn't mean lose weight or be as light as possible. It means staying at an appropriate weight for what you want to achieve athletically. You want to be strong enough to handle the demands of your sport and light enough to not place undue stress on your joints. You'll know you're at a good weight when you regularly feel capable, powerful, and energetic when exercising.

Body over mind:

Common advice for athletes under duress is "mind over body." We're told we'll only reach our potential if we "push through the pain." And that's true (if clichéd) if we're talking about something like slacking off the pace or doing fewer reps simply because we're feeling tired.

But in terms of avoiding injury, "mind over body" is horrible advice. You're not a robot. If there's a conflict between what your training program says you should do and what your body is telling you, in the form of acute, site-specific pain, listen to your body.

Be a full-time athlete:

This doesn't mean to shirk your everyday responsibilities and obsess over your workouts. But remain conscious of the fact that what you do in the many hours a day you're not exercising affects the time when you are working out. What you eat, how you deal with stress, how you sit, how much you sit, and many other seemingly small matters can detract from the quality and quantity of your training.

One of the most important matters in this regard is the least active—your sleep. In the next chapter, we'll look at how CBD can help your workouts by improving your sleep.

Key Points on CBD and Athletic Injuries

- Athletes increasingly recognize the limitations and dangers of prescription pain medication and conventional over-the-counter analgesics.
- Research and anecdotal evidence support the idea that CBD can lower site-specific inflammation and pain.
- CBD appears to be most effective in managing overuse injuries involving tendons, ligaments, and joints.
- During and after treating injuries with CBD, address the underlying issues so that the injury doesn't return.

Chapter 5

CBD and Better Sleep

If you're old enough, you might remember when hotels catered to business travelers with promises of exciting entertainment and late-hours partying. Now they coddle you with in-room chamomile tea, blackout shades, and other aids to that most elusive of travel companions: a good night's sleep.

It's not just travelers who pine for peaceful slumber. High-quality sleep of decent duration is one of the most prized accomplishments of modern life. In a National Sleep Foundation survey, 45 percent of Americans said that poor-quality sleep interferes with their daily activities at least one day a week. The Centers for Disease Control and Prevention (CDC) has reported that one-third of Americans regularly get less than the suggested minimum of seven hours of sleep per day.

Despite the national longing for better sleep, people seem to enjoy telling others how little they sleep. The tales often have an undertone that equates not sleeping much with being more productive. The facts about sleep deprivation say otherwise, at least if you care about the quality of what you're doing during all that time awake.

There's no universal necessary amount of sleep, which makes it easier for people to convince themselves they're getting enough. That said, most adults do best with between seven and nine hours of sleep per day.

In the short term, sleep deprivation leads to impaired cognitive function, memory, and alertness, even after just one night of inadequate sleep. It's been shown to double the risk for on-the-job injuries and is estimated to contribute to at least 100,000 car crashes and more than 1,500 fatalities a year. More subjectively, sleep deprivation leads to being more impulsive, irritable, indecisive, clumsy, and hungry.

Long-term sleep deprivation has serious health consequences, including an increased risk for high blood pressure, stroke, heart disease, immune system compromise, obesity, arthritis, and depression. Research on mortality and long-term sleep deprivation has found that people who report getting less than six or seven hours per day are at a greater risk of dying in a given period.

CBD's entry into the mainstream is due in large part to its reputation for helping with sleep. The number of people who have ever said, "I wish I didn't sleep as well" is exactly zero. That's especially true of athletes, who need good sleep not only to meet their workaday responsibilities but also to be at their physical and psychological best when working out.

Why Sleep Is So Important for Athletes

If the above isn't enough to convince you of the need for consistent good sleep, think about your workouts. Research on Stanford University athletes has found a direct relationship between better sleep and physical performance. Swimmers who increased their sleep time improved their reaction time, kick rate, and sprint times. Basketball players also were faster sprinters, and were more accurate free-throw shooters, when they started sleeping better. These improvements suggest the athletes' central nervous systems were operating at a higher level, an athlete's version of overcoming the clumsiness that often accompanies sleep deprivation.

If you care more about endurance performance, there's evidence that, while short-term sleep deprivation might not decrease your aerobic capacity, it does increase your perceived exertion at a given workload. That is, you might swim your laps or run your neighborhood course at the same pace, but doing so will feel harder. There's also the subjective matter of being less willing to push or persevere when you're sleep deprived. That phenomenon can indirectly lower your fitness if you regularly cut workouts short or back off on intensity because you're feeling zonked.

In addition to poor performance or low motivation, there's also injury. A Brown University study of collegiate cross-country runners found that those who reported poor-quality sleep were significantly more likely to get injured during their three-month season than those who reported better sleep. The difference remained even when other predictors of injury, such as increasing training by too much and having a preseason injury, were accounted for.

Overall, athletes have a leg up on sedentary people, because regular exercise is known to improve sleep quality. But there can be sport-specific challenges. You're probably familiar with the tired-but-wired feeling after an exceptionally long and/or intense workout. This happens because your nervous and hormonal systems are overstimulated. While they try to bring your body back to homeostasis, they can disrupt your sleep, which is, of course, one of the best ways to get back to normal.

Logistically, getting enough sleep can be difficult for everyday athletes because there are only so many hours in a day. Morning exercise usually means getting up earlier than you otherwise would. If you work out after work, you might need to exercise closer to bedtime than is recommended. Or maybe you exercise right after work, but by the time you get home and tend to your responsibilities there, you wind up having dinner late, which can interfere with getting to sleep at a decent hour (or staying asleep once you're in bed).

If you're sleep deprived, you probably know it. Even if you think you're not, ask yourself: Do I fall asleep almost instantly? Do I doze off in dark environments, such as a movie theater, during daylight hours? Other signs include relying on an alarm clock to wake, feeling sleepy when driving, relying on caffeine to get through your days, difficulty focusing your eyes, and not feeling rested when you get out of bed.

How CBD Might Improve Your Sleep

To understand how CBD might help with sleep, and why other common sleep aids might be worth avoiding, it helps to know a little about what happens when we sleep. There are four stages of sleep. One of the four is rapid-eye-movement (REM) sleep; the other three are non-REM sleep. A normal sleep cycle progresses through the four stages. In healthy sleep, you will go through each stage to complete one cycle and will have five to six cycles per overall sleep period.

Stage 1 is the transition period between being awake and deeper sleep. Bodily functions such as heart rate, breathing, and brain activity start to slow. This period, known as sleep onset latency, should be the shortest of the four, about 10 to 20 minutes. As noted above, one sign of chronic sleep deprivation is falling asleep almost immediately when given the opportunity. On the other hand, what's known as poor sleep hygiene—such as going to bed overstimulated from caffeine, phone use, or anxiety—can make stage 1 frustratingly long.

In stage 2, you're fully asleep and your body temperature has dropped, but you aren't yet sleeping deeply. It's relatively easy to wake someone in stage 2. In a normal sleep cycle, you spend more time in this stage than in each of the others.

Stage 3 is the deepest period of sleep, and essential to good health and athletic performance. Tissue repair, bone and muscle building, and immune system strengthening happen during stage 3. (Figuratively, it's the stuff of dreams, given all the good things that happen during it, although technically stage 4 is the dreamy one.) If you've ever been woken and felt briefly disoriented, you were probably in stage 3.

In stage 4, REM sleep, the slowed breathing and heart rate of stages 2 and 3 accelerate. This is REM sleep, when dreams occur. In a healthy sleep cycle, you'll first hit stage 4 about 90 minutes after falling asleep, and you'll stay in it the first time for about 10 minutes. Then you'll spend more time in stage 4 each time you reach it, so that by the time you wake for good you'll have spent about 20 percent of your total sleep time in stage 4.

Given the widespread sleep problems noted at the beginning of this chapter, many Americans often don't sleep this way. They struggle to fall asleep, they struggle to stay asleep, they struggle to get out of bed when they need to because the intended four-stage cycles are so out of whack. One sign of the severity of the problem: A CDC survey earlier this decade found that 4 percent of American adults had taken a prescription sleep medication in the previous month.

If you've suffered through chronic poor sleep, you can't begrudge people for turning to prescription sleep meds, also known as hypnotics. But the evidence against them is overwhelmingly negative, on two main fronts. First, as described in a 2016 review of hypnotics by Daniel Kripke, MD, a seminal sleep researcher, the drugs are associated with all sorts of bad health outcomes, including increased risk of cancer, infections, depression, accidents, and even death. The drugs can also worsen insomnia once people stop taking them. Second, all these costs come without much benefit. A large review of clinical trials found that the most common class of prescription drugs (including brands like Ambien and Zolpimist) reduced sleep latency by an average of 12 minutes, but increased total sleep time by only 11 minutes. Some research has found that this class of drugs doesn't increase the percentage of time spent in stage 3, the restorative period of sleep so important to athletes.

So it's not surprising that more people, especially athletes, are looking for alternatives. How might CBD help?

Consider first the general sense. "Think about CBD allowing things to happen rather than causing things to happen," says Sanjeev Javia, a veteran developer of hemp products and other plant-based supplements. "In terms of sleep, that means what's needed by the body for it to happen. CBD is there to provide balance—when the body gets calmed down, it can relax and unwind and do the things that allow sleep to happen."

This is a different outlook than the "take pill = fall asleep" model of prescription medications. "It's not getting the end product of sleep, but getting the body to where the body can get the product," Javia says.

Philip Blair, MD, sounds a similar note. "Sleep quality appears to be directly related to a healthy endocannabinoid system," he says. "It's kind of a game of connect the dots—if you restore balance to that system, then, by virtue of its effect on sleep quality, you'll get more of that deep, restful, restorative sleep."

There's not as much research as would be ideal on how CBD might connect those dots. A review of studies on cannabis, cannabinoids, and sleep published in 2017 concluded, "Research on cannabis and sleep is in its infancy and has yielded mixed results."

There are some leads, though, from animal and human research. Perhaps the most intriguing findings from animal studies have to do with rats and slow-wave sleep; the latter is the rodent equivalent of our stage 3 sleep, the restorative period that's so crucial to athletes. Research has found that CBD both shortens the amount of time it takes for rats to attain slow-wave sleep and increases the amount of time rats spend in that phase.

In humans, research published in 2019 by the Kaiser-Permanente health insurance company looked at the effect of 25 milligrams a day of CBD on 72 adults. Of them, 47 said their primary complaint was anxiety, and the other 25 said their main concern was poor sleep. Despite the differing motivations for taking CBD, there appeared to be crossover benefits. Nearly 80 percent of the people in the study, including some of those who were seeking help with sleep, said their anxiety levels decreased during the three-month study period. Two-thirds of the participants reported that their sleep improved within the first month of starting to take CBD.

These findings mesh with research published almost four decades ago. People who sought treatment at a sleep clinic for insomnia reported better sleep and less dream recall with regular CBD use. The finding on dream recall could mean that one aspect of sleeping better was waking less often—think about how much easier it is to remember a bad dream when you get up right after it ends, compared to those vague memories hours later.

Another link between CBD and REM sleep: usually while you're dreaming, your muscles are temporarily paralyzed. That's good, because it keeps you from acting out the dreams playing out in your mind. In people with REM sleep disorder, that paralysis sometimes doesn't happen. You flail and twitch and otherwise move around, and sometimes scream, all of which means you wake feeling less refreshed. A small study published in 2014 found that Parkinson's patients with this disorder experienced near-immediate relief from their symptoms when they started taking CBD.

There's also preliminary evidence that cannabis might reduce the time it takes to fall asleep, but some of that research has been on THC only, and some has been on THC combined with CBD.

Not all human sleep research has been pro-CBD. A Brazilian study found no difference in the amount of time spent in each of the four phases of sleep, or subjects' subjective reports of how well they slept, when they took 300 milligrams of CBD or a placebo half an hour before going to bed. That seems like a significant finding, especially considering that 300 milligrams is 10 to 20 times as much as many people take in a typical presleep dose.

Then again, maybe it's not all that significant when you realize the study looked at these factors for only two nights, one when taking CBD and one when taking the placebo. There's also the caveat necessary for any short-term sleep study done in a lab—in addition to the variable being tested (here, CBD or placebo), there's the unknown factor of how the unfamiliar environment affected the subjects' sleep.

It's not really helpful to think of CBD as the cannabis equivalent to Ambien or other hypnotics. Honest advocates of CBD for sleep don't claim predictable benefits on an acute basis. The idea is that, over time, you'll more often than not realize you're sleeping better and waking feeling more refreshed.

The idea of subtle change over time should be familiar

to athletes. If you commit to stretching after every workout, it's unlikely that on the first day of doing so you'll notice a difference. But after a month, you'll probably realize you feel a little less creaky at the start of workouts and more fluid while exercising. The same idea applies to other things we do as athletes, such as improving our diets or staying on top of hydration.

Or you might notice CBD's effect on your sleep only in its absence. Chase Knight, a CrossFit instructor from Kansas City, Missouri, doesn't consistently take CBD because of the cost. "While on it, I didn't think I felt all that different," he says, "but about a week after I stopped taking it, I started having brain farts throughout the day, and was waking up more tired." A military veteran, Knight wrestles with insomnia and sleep apnea. "I usually wake two to five times a night, and I'm usually groggy when I get out of bed," he says. "I realized when I stopped taking CBD that, while on it, I was up less frequently, and when I woke during the night, I got back to sleep more quickly."

Several athletes I spoke with said they noticed improved sleep as an unexpected side benefit when they started taking CBD. Professional triathlete Andrew Talansky, of Napa, California, turned to CBD for help with recovery from hard training and anxiety about his transition from cycling to a new sport. "The first thing I noticed—within a week—was that I was sleeping better," he says. Another triathlete, Carol Pope, of San Antonio, Texas, initially investigated CBD for help with low-back pain from long bike rides. Now she's made an oral spray part of her prebed routine and says she plans to take CBD indefinitely, in part because of how it helps her sleep.

As I mentioned before, I came to CBD with the primary hope that it would improve my sleep and therefore help me feel better running. A little personal report on the matter:

Partly owing to dysthymia, or chronic low-grade depression, I've often had poor-quality sleep. It's typical for me to wake often and then get psychologically stuck—rehashing a perceived slight from the previous day, dreading the seemingly endless chores that await me after sunrise, or, on the worst nights, despairing over the pointlessness of existence itself. These stare-at-the-ceiling interludes can last an hour or more. I've sometimes welcomed being sick, because then I could justify taking something like Nyquil and count on being zonked out.

So when I started hearing more and more reports that other middle-aged ruminators were taking CBD to help with sleep, I was intrigued. I wasn't even thinking about my athletic life. I just wanted to see if I could have fewer dark nights of the soul.

I started sleeping better within the first week of taking prebed CBD. I still wake more frequently than I'd like, but the difference in how I usually feel when I do is profound. My norm used to be concern for how unrefreshed I felt and concern that I'd feel no better when it was time to get out of bed. Now, more often than not, I think, "If I had to get up for good now, I'd be okay." Sometimes when I feel this way I'll look at the time and see that I've been asleep for only a few hours. That realization sets off a positive feedback loop—if I go back to sleep quickly, I tell myself, I'll feel that much more rested in the morning. When the darker thoughts do creep in, it has become easier to practice mindfulness techniques and other cognitive tricks to return to sleep. It's rare that I now wake groggy and dragging. I more often feel like I did as a teen, when I would leave bed eager to go for a run and other enjoyable parts of the day. My summation when someone asks: I don't sleep longer since starting to take CBD, I sleep better.

That last point is crucial for time-pressed athletes. Many of us work out early in the morning because we can count on fewer obstacles and interruptions at that time of day. That claimed time can come with a price, namely, skimping on sleep. If this is your reality, you've no doubt had mornings when you greet the alarm by wondering if, overall, you'd be better skipping your workout and getting more sleep. If CBD improves your sleep, you'll still have to get up early to exercise, but you'll probably do so feeling more refreshed.

"Whether you work nine to five or are a pro athlete, you have to wake up in the morning and perform," says Riley Cote, a former NHL player who now owns the CBD brand BodyChek Wellness. "When you sleep better, everything becomes better. Getting good sleep is key to a preventative approach to your health as an athlete, rather than being reactive and being like, 'Oh crap, now I'm injured, now I'm burnt out, let me throw a bunch of sleep meds and pain meds at the problem.'"

How to Maximize CBD's Sleep Enhancement Benefits

Every expert I talked with on the subject of CBD and sleep made some version of this point: you're wasting your money if you take CBD but otherwise continue to do things that interfere with good sleep. "CBD's not a magic bullet," says Karyemaitre Aliffe, MD. "That's a mechanical model—that there's a button in the body you can push to make this one thing happen. That's a very linear model. The body is built on systems, and systems are nonlinear."

There are two main topics to address in this realm. The first—and most common, and easier to fix—is your presleep routine and environment.

Reduce evening use of electronic screens:

Let's start with perhaps the major impediment to good sleep, even though it wasn't a problem until recently. Yes, I'm talking about your phone. Depending on what survey you read, somewhere between two-thirds and three-quarters of American adults say they go to bed with their phone within reach, with the proportion even greater in people under the age of 30.

One issue is the just-one-more-text phenomenon that can mean staying up later than you otherwise would. Regardless of if you're looking at friends' photos or getting riled up over politics, your brain is engaged and stimulated. Think about how much easier it is to fall asleep when you're calm and relaxed versus dealing with a racing mind. It's also tempting to grab your bedside phone during the night to check the time or look for new notifications. Doing so will inform you at the cost of interrupted sleep.

More specific to phones, tablets, laptops, and the like, the blue light that these gadgets emit is at a wavelength that interferes with your body's secretion of melatonin, a hormone that helps to regulate your circadian rhythms. Exposure to blue light in the evening has been shown to delay the release of melatonin, with the result that your body thinks it's not yet time to fall asleep. Then, once you do fall asleep, your body secretes melatonin later than it otherwise would, and you can wake feeling groggy.

Try keeping phones and other devices with screens, including televisions, out of your bedroom. If you're not sleeping better after a week or two, take the next step and institute a curfew—no gadget use in the hour before you plan to go to bed.

Make your bedroom dark, quiet, and cool:

A screen-free bedroom is a great first step for building the right environment for sleep. Quiet and darkness are obvious next steps. When your body's natural sleep cycle is allowed to happen, your body temperature will start to drop as bedtime approaches. You can help this phenomenon do its thing by having your bedroom a little cooler than the rest of your living space.

Establish a prebed routine:

As an athlete, you probably have a pre-exercise routine that helps set you up for a successful workout. Apply that approach to the time before you go to bed. Know what your too-late times for caffeine and alcohol are, and stick to them. Prepare your body and mind for sleep with practices you might do as part of a postworkout cooldown, such as gentle stretching or yoga poses and breathing exercises.

And, of course, consider making CBD a part of your prebed routine. Take tinctures within the hour before you hope to fall asleep, either solo or added to something else that can help you fall asleep, such as herbal tea or warm milk. If you take CBD in capsule form, consume it more like one to two hours before bedtime, to account for a longer digestion process.

The second topic to address to complement CBD's effectiveness is nonenvironmental impediments to good sleep.

Address the emotional issues that are keeping you awake:

"When we talk about insomnia and other sleep problems, we seldom ask 'why,'" Aliffe says. "Why are you in this situation in the first place? Are you excited, frustrated, depressed? CBD or prescription sleep drugs don't resolve that issue. If you're worried about something and that's why you're having trouble sleeping, you would benefit from scaling back on the thing that's causing worry *and* taking CBD. If you just throw CBD at the problem, you might wind up more worried. You might think, 'I took CBD, it's supposed to help me sleep, but I'm not sleeping any better. What's wrong with me?'"

Address the physical issues that are keeping you awake:

That thinking also applies to physical obstacles to good sleep. If you have an athletic injury that wakes you, figure out how to get healthy again. On any given day, you might not be sufficiently recovered from your workouts—your muscles might be twitchy or pulsing, your back might be sore, your nervous and hormonal systems might be out of whack and working overtime when they should be relaxed.

Sleep is an important aspect of recovery from training and competition, but not the only one. We'll turn to the bigger picture of recovery in the next chapter.

Key Points on CBD and Sleep

- Good sleep is crucial to your overall health and athletic performance.
- Prescription sleep medications are associated with significant health risks while barely increasing sleep time.
- CBD appears to help many people fall asleep faster and spend more time in slow-wave sleep, during which muscle repair and other important aspects of recovering from training occur.
- Many athletes find that CBD helps them sleep better, not longer.
- Create a good sleep environment to maximize CBD's sleep benefits.

Chapter 6

CBD and Recovery

In one sense, this whole book is about CBD and recovery.

Athletic recovery essentially means restoring balance in your body after exercise. (That's balance in the sense of systemic harmony, not how whether you can stand on one foot while putting on your socks.) A more technical word for balance is *homeostasis,* or stable equilibrium between your body's interdependent systems. If the endocannabinoid system is responsible for maintaining homeostasis, and if CBD improves the functioning of the endocannabinoid system, then all of the specific benefits claimed for CBD—better sleep, lower inflammation, calmer mental state, and so on— are really just subsets of the overall concept of recovery.

At the same time, athletes have a more specific concept of recovery. We mean the process of getting our body back to its pre-exercise state so that we can absorb the benefits of the workout we just did and be ready for the next one. That's the sense in which we'll look at CBD and recovery in this chapter.

Why Recovery Is Key to Performance

"I once asked an NFL coach about the differences among pro football players," says Sanjeev Javia, a veteran developer of hemp products and other plant-based supplements. "How much better are the ones that get the most play time? He said that most are roughly the same in terms of their capabilities. What distinguishes the ones who play more is that they're better at recovery. They're the ones most able to be there performing at the highest level most often."

Javia's anecdote is a good way to think about your own athletic life—not in the context of comparison to other athletes but in the context of comparison to various versions of yourself. Consider those days when everything feels great and you go farther or faster or do more reps than usual. You probably think of those days as flukes. "Where did that come from?" you might ask yourself.

A great workout isn't a fluke. By definition, you can't do something you're not capable of. A great workout or competition is a glimpse of your potential. You can more often and more deeply tap into your full potential—and you can more fully develop your potential—by getting recovery right. To understand what this entails, let's step back and briefly consider what happens when you work out.

Challenging workouts provide a stimulus for your body to improve in some way, such as building more muscle or increasing your aerobic capacity. For example, when you lift weights to failure, your body thinks, "Hmm, she might do this again, I better be ready next time," and creates more and stronger muscle fibers. As you're probably well aware, in the immediate aftermath of a hard workout, you don't feel fitter. You feel tired. You're quite unlikely to be able to lift more weight, or run faster, or ride farther the day after a workout that pushes your limits. But if you allow the stress-adaptation process to run its course, you'll get fitter.

Recovery is allowing that process to happen. The key to getting the biggest fitness gains isn't to work out hard; almost anybody can do that on any one day. The key is to manage your recovery in such a way that you can regularly do those challenging workouts. After all, a single workout, no matter how draining, does little to make you fitter. It's the steady accumulation of those workouts that leads to the real gains. Good recovery allows you to do those workouts more often and/or do them at a higher level of quality.

Even if you have no competitive or other performance goals, recovery is key to a satisfying athletic life. Who wouldn't rather feel fresh and eager rather than stale and apathetic most days? Good recovery simply makes exercising more enjoyable, which makes consistency more likely, which leads to greater fitness. Recovering well from your workouts also means that you'll feel more lively in the several hours a day when you're not working out.

There's great variability among athletes in recovery rates. Big-picture contributing factors include genetics, age, fitness level, training history, lifestyle, and gender. (Women tend to recover more slowly than men because of lower testosterone levels.) This is why it can be tricky to train frequently with the same person. Even if you're more or less as fit as each other, your friend might be ready for another long or hard workout after one recovery day, while you might be better off with two easy days.

There's also great variability within your own ability to recover. The most obvious example is over a long time—because of factors such as changes in hormone levels and injury history, you probably can't mimic the workout schedule of your 20s when you're in your 50s. But your ability to recover can also change greatly over shorter periods. If you're swamped at work and dealing with a family crisis and having trouble sleeping, you'll likely take longer to recover than when things are calm.

Several workout-related factors can influence your short-term recovery rate. Depleting your body's stored form of carbohydrate, glycogen, is one aim of long runs, rides, and swims. Doing so increases your body's ability to store glycogen, thereby improving your endurance. But in the immediate aftermath of one of these long workouts, you need to rebuild your glycogen stores, which can take 24 hours or longer, depending on how depleted you got and how well you refueled. Hard and/or long workouts also temporarily suppress your immune system. In the few hours to even few days after one of these sessions, you're at greater risk of infection. Microscopic muscle tears, usually stemming from unaccustomed activities or excessive pounding, can lead to delayed-onset muscle soreness (DOMS), which tends to peak 24 to 48 hours after the workout that caused it. Going long or hard again while "enjoying" DOMS, or while your immune system is suppressed, or while your glycogen stores are depleted, usually results in subpar workouts and greater recovery time from the initial workout.

There's also a subjective aspect to recovery. When you feel chronically subpar, you're less likely to push when it's time to push. The same is true if your workout routine feels monotonous. You can be fine physically, but if you're psychologically fatigued your training will be compromised.

How CBD Might Help with Recovery

Where does CBD fit into all of this? As you can see from the above, your response to training is a complex, subtle interplay among many factors, both physical and psychological. Your endocannabinoid system plays a crucial role in managing that process because of its involvement in things like how you react to stress, your mood, your sleep, your immune system, your metabolism, and your hormonal system. So if CBD helps your endocannabinoid system work optimally, then it should help with restoring homeostasis after your workouts.

Unfortunately, there's basically no published research on CBD and athletic recovery. Two reasons: First, as we've seen, there's little research on CBD and exercise in general. Second, even if there were, the broad concept of "recovery" is difficult to study following typical research protocols. Studies focus on specific variables. Traditional anti-inflammatory medications have been found to lower muscle soreness and swelling in studies that induce DOMS. In separate studies, massage has been found to achieve similar results. But in both cases, the subjects' muscle function improved no more than that of people not receiving those treatments. So did the anti-inflammatories or massage really speed recovery? That's harder to say.

We've seen in previous chapters how CBD might lower inflammation and improve sleep, two important aspects of good recovery. In the following chapter we'll look at the evidence for CBD reducing stress and anxiety. Help in those areas should also contribute to faster recovery—these benefits can work together in a 1 + 1 + 1 = 5 fashion.

That synergy is certainly what you hear when athletes talk about CBD and recovery. A subjective sense of feeling better able to get back out there the day after a hard workout, not feeling as fatigued several hours after a workout, and overall spryness are common reports. The owner of one CBD company said to me of its primarily middle-aged customers, "They'll do a long, hard workout on Sunday. They tell us, 'I'm not as sore, I don't need to lie on the couch all day because I'm so beat up and tired, and the next day I can go to work and function at a higher level.' Or we hear from people that they go on a week-long ski trip and can ski hard every day."

Ashley Mayer, a naturopathic doctor in Scottsdale, Arizona, says that she recommends CBD "for my intense athletes or people who still want to continue to be athletes when things start to break down." Mayer says it helps these athletes' muscle soreness, and she adds, "Generally, my clientele who are into sports are Type A, highly active people who tend to have anxiety and insomnia issues, so CBD around bedtime for them is good because it will help them with recovery."

Here are other athletes' reports on CBD and recovery.

Will Eaton: A former special operations member of the Marine Corps, Eaton now works in sales in Arvada, Colorado. He does half and full Ironman triathlons, half marathons and marathons, mountain bike races, and, annually, the Pikes Peak Ascent, a 13.3-mile race up the 14,000-footer.

"I'm the idiot who you call on a Wednesday and ask, 'Will you run a half marathon with me on Saturday?' and I always say yes," Eaton jokes.

Eaton began taking CBD in 2017, around the time he turned 40. "I wouldn't say it's done much for my sleep," he says. "The benefits I see are that I don't get as sore and my recovery is faster. In the past, the next morning I was in the pain cave. Now I can more often get out there the next day and do something ambitious."

Justin Diamond: A triathlete in college, Diamond switched to professional road cycling after graduation, then more recently transitioned to adventure cycling. In the summer of 2018, he was part of a small group that rode the entirety of Route 66, roughly 2,500 miles from Chicago to Los Angeles, in 26 days.

Diamond started hearing about CBD from fellow cyclists in 2017. "I thought, 'I don't want to get high,'" he says. "Then I did my research and got on board. I wanted to stop taking Advil but wanted that relief."

During the Route 66 ride, Diamond upped his usual CBD intake to speed recovery. He took a 25-milligram capsule and drank a protein powder with CBD right after finishing riding for the day and took another 25-milligram capsule before going to bed.

Two of the other riders took CBD from the start. A few others on the journey were skeptical. "But then when they started to get achy and worn down, and we seemed to be recovering better, they wanted to try it," Diamond says. "Within a couple days they started feeling better, and their knee and Achilles aches improved."

Lexi duPont: A professional mountain free-skier, duPont

has placed as high as third in the Freeskiing World Tour. Her nonskiing activities include sailing, biking, surfing, climbing, hiking, and yoga.

She learned about CBD from some cousins, who told her it would help with inflammation, muscle recovery, sleep, and anxiety. "I have always been a big believer in the healing benefits of plant-based medicine," duPont says. "I was over-taking Advil and Tylenol and loading myself up on caffeine in the morning. I quickly discovered CBD could do all of that and more without the long-term side effects."

DuPont typically takes a few droppers of a full-spectrum tincture before going to bed. But she's not tied to a set amount. "When you take big slams or ouch your adrenal glands to the max, recovery is everything," she says. "Every day is different, and I give my body what it wants."

Greg Kogut: A road cyclist in his mid-40s from San Diego, Kogut has one of the more interesting CBD stories I've heard. He learned about CBD from reading several articles and was intrigued enough to do his own research. He wound up spending six months trying different dosages of different potencies of tinctures (from 250 milligrams to 1,250 milligrams of CBD per 1-ounce bottle).

His experience was . . . inconclusive. "I can't say that it has any recovery, performance, or anti-inflammatory benefit," Kogut says. "Nor can I say it doesn't do things. I had no noticeable alterations in my training. I have no acute injuries I'm dealing with. So there was going to be no magic cure for me."

The exception: Kogut found that at the higher range of dosage he experimented with, CBD had a relaxing effect on him, "almost to the point of drowsiness," he says. "After very intense races I'm sort of wired and irritable for a day or two. I think it may have helped with that." (That wired-but-tired feeling is a classic sign of the adrenal glands and nervous system working overtime.) Kogut now uses CBD only after races or very intense workouts to help return his body to homeostasis.

Finally, me: As I said in the previous chapter, the first thing I noticed when I started taking CBD was improved sleep. The second was, for lack of a better term, less overall creakiness. I'm in my mid-50s and am relatively pain-free, but more than 100,000 miles of running over the last four decades are going to leave their mark. In my second week of taking CBD, I found I was a little more lively getting out of bed, a little less beaten up hours after running. This subtle improvement leads not only to being able to run a little farther and faster but wanting to do so. Or if I don't want to train more ambitiously, it makes whatever mix of volume and intensity I do more enjoyable.

My usual CBD routine is a prebed dropper of tincture plus topicals as warranted. The main exception is after my longest and/or hardest workouts, which are always in the morning. I'll have an additional serving of CBD soon after those runs, usually mixed in with food or drink I consume within the first hour of finishing. I seem to not feel as zonked in the afternoon when I do that. I still do just easy running the following day, but those runs are now less often a when-will-this-be-over slog, and my overall energy level for the rest of my life is higher. To me, that means recovery.

How to Maximize CBD's Help with Recovery

There's definitely a synergy involved in recovery. The more you do besides take CBD, the better off you'll be. Here are some other recovery best practices.

Do a cooldown after hard workouts:

Stretching or other flexibility work is adequate after most workouts. (More on that below.) After harder sessions, such as interval training or sustained faster-than-usual workouts, a cooldown will more quickly return your body to its pre-workout state.

Ten to 15 minutes at a very light intensity of the activity you just did will increase blood flow, which will speed the removal of waste products from your muscles and blood; reduce hormone levels, which will help your metabolism return to normal sooner; and reduce your chances of developing DOMS. If you can't stand another step of running or another pedal stroke or lap in the pool, gentle versions of other aerobic activities will achieve the same purpose. Swimmers might spin on a bike for 15 minutes, runners might kick in a pool, cyclists might go for a walk, and so on.

Do some gentle flexibility work:

There are no studies proving that stretching after exercise prevents injury. There's a ton of anecdotal evidence, however, that 5 to 10 minutes of gentle flexibility work when your muscles are warmed and loose will help you feel better at the start of your next workout.

Stretching and yoga are the obvious go-tos here but are

not the only options. Technique drills and mobility exercises such as clamshells and leg lifts are viable choices. Foam rolling your chronic sore spots at this time is also helpful.

Change clothes:

I don't mean to sound like your mother here, but put on some dry clothes! This is especially good advice if you've driven to your workout and won't be home for a while. I know several people who, on a cold day, have delayed their recovery after a long run by standing around chatting, then running errands, and then eventually getting home to change out of their damp workout outfit. A day or two later they find they're dragging more than should be the case.

Compression tights and knee-high socks are good choices after your hardest or longest workouts. There's decent evidence that these garments reduce DOMS and perceived fatigue.

Take in fluids:

During exercise, drinking to thirst is usually adequate to prevent significant dehydration. After exercise, however, your thirst mechanism can be blunted. Rehydrating quickly is essential to restoring cellular homeostasis. So you might need to be disciplined about drinking enough if you've sweated a lot.

Aim to take in 150 percent of the fluids you lose in sweat (e.g., drink 24 ounces if you lost a pound [16 ounces] during your workout). That's enough to account for some of what you'll lose as urine.

Water is always a good choice for immediate rehydration. Other beverages are useful after that first round of drinking if you tend not to drink enough plain water. Sodium in drinks helps you to retain more of the fluid you take in and can spur consuming more. This is also a good time for flavored or flavor-free CBD powders.

Take in calories:

Long aerobic workouts (90 minutes or longer) will drain your body's glycogen stores. Muscles restock those stores at a higher rate in the first two hours, and especially in the first 30 minutes, after a long, draining workout. A carbohydrate-to-protein ratio of 3:1 or 4:1 will further speed glycogen resynthesis.

If your stomach is too upset to eat during this soon-after window, recovery drinks or smoothies are a good choice. You can easily add CBD powder to liquid calories.

Have variety in your training:

Follow your longest and hardest workout days with days of reduced volume and intensity. Easy days are not the time to stare at your GPS watch or power meter and strain to reach a certain level of performance. These are the days when you're most fatigued. Pushing harder on these days than what feels comfortable won't make you tougher or fitter. Doing so will just make you more tired and sore and prolong the time until you're ready to do the more challenging workouts that really advance your fitness.

Make your easy days even more restorative by minimizing the stress on your muscles and nervous system. Stick with activities that won't encourage more DOMS; for example, if your legs are sore from a long bike ride, don't make your easy riding day the day you really hit the leg weights. If you run, seek flat, level, soft surfaces, which will be gentler on your muscles, joints, and bones.

Sleep well:
You'll remember from the previous chapter that your body repairs itself during slow-wave sleep. Do what you can, perhaps including taking CBD, to increase the amount of time you spend in that sleep phase.

Key Points on CBD and Recovery

- Recovery entails bringing your body back into balance as soon as possible after challenging workouts.
- Although specific physiological processes are involved, recovery is best understood as a body-wide phenomenon.
- CBD can help athletic recovery by more quickly returning the body to preworkout equilibrium.
- A few simple other recovery practices can enhance CBD's effectiveness.

Chapter 7

CBD and Athletic Anxiety

It's estimated that almost 30 percent of Americans will develop an anxiety disorder at some point in their life. Everyone worries about things at times; that's not anxiety any more than getting down when things aren't going well is depression. Anxiety is more nebulous, a general sense of unease and worry, often accompanied by physical symptoms like increased heart rate and sweating that are associated with the body's fight-or-flight mechanism.

Although exercise is a great way to manage chronic and acute anxiety, athletes aren't immune. We tend to be driven, goal-oriented people. These traits help us to accomplish more than we otherwise would, but they can also too easily spill over into unhelpful thoughts and behaviors. In fact, in addition to the types and targets of anxiety that everyone else is subject to, athletes can get anxious about training and competition, which should be antidotes to everyday stress.

"Anxiety can ruin your life no matter how healthy and fit you are," says Karyemaitre Aliffe, MD. That's why

Aliffe and other medical advocates of cannabis are so keen on CBD's potential to provide sustained relief from anxiety.

Stress and the Endocannabinoid System

One way of thinking about anxiety is that it's the result of the body's stress response malfunctioning. That's true whether the stress—which a 2010 *Journal of Neuroscience* overview defined as "any stimulus that presents a challenge to homeostasis"—is real or imagined.

When such a challenge is perceived, the part of your brain called the hypothalamus releases hormones. These chemicals reach the pituitary gland and stimulate the release of other hormones. These, in turn, cause the adrenal glands to release cortisol, the so-called "stress hormone." Cortisol prompts responses from various bodily systems (cardiovascular, metabolic, immune, and others) that prepare you to best deal with the stress.

This stress-response system is a normal—and useful!—bodily function. Problems arise when the system goes awry, such as swinging into action too often, or out of proportion to threats, or inappropriately. Chronic overstimulation can severely harm your physical and mental health.

There's increasing consensus that the endocannabinoid system plays a key role in managing stress response. Endocannabinoids regulate the amount and frequency of the hormones released by the hypothalamus that kick off the fight-or-flight mechanism. When your endocannabinoid levels are out of whack, your stress response might be triggered too readily. Or your stress response might not be as easily inhibited when what was initially perceived as a challenge turns out to be a nonissue. (Think about that jolt of adrenaline you might get from a near accident when driving, and how quickly the surge usually dissipates when you realize you're okay.)

The endocannabinoid system also helps to manage chronic stress. First, if it's well-functioning, it can alter your immediate reaction to a regular stressor, such that your body doesn't go into overdrive every time it encounters a challenging situation it's dealt with before. Second, and related, endocannabinoids within the part of the brain called the amygdala help to control cognitive and emotional responses to stress. This process can help to keep anxiety from spiking despite the body's signals that a challenge is present. This higher-level management of stress can also help to mold memories of challenging situations so that they don't take as great of a toll.

It's a pretty simple—and logical—step to take to say that if a well-functioning endocannabinoid system is key to managing anxiety, and if CBD can improve the functioning of the endocannabinoid system, then CBD can help to manage anxiety.

Research supports this line of thinking. In a study published in *Neuropsychopharmacology* in 2004, people's moods were assessed and their brains were imaged on separate occasions, once after taking CBD and once after taking a placebo. After they took CBD, the subjects reported decreased anxiety. This subjective result coincided with anxiety-lowering activity in the hypothalamus, amygdala, and other parts of the brain. Other studies have found that CBD can significantly affect cortisol levels and can lower subjective symptoms of anxiety when taken before a typically stressful situation. Animal studies have shown CBD to work on the parts of the brain involved in forming memories of stressful situations, so that encountering the situation again doesn't automatically produce an anxious response.

One key potential pathway: CBD might work similarly to one main class of modern antidepressant medications. Called selective serotonin reuptake inhibitors (SSRIs), these drugs are often prescribed to treat anxiety. Serotonin and other neurotransmitters are associated with mood regulation. SSRIs are thought to work by keeping serotonin in the space between brain cells for longer, rather than being immediately reabsorbed (that's the "reuptake inhibitor" part of the name). "There's legitimate evidence of CBD working on serotonin receptors," says Scott Palmer, MD. "That's why you hear a lot of people saying that CBD has a calming effect—the stimulation of serotonin with CBD can help with mood, anxiety, and depression."

How CBD Might Help with Athletic Anxiety

Exercise is increasingly recognized as an effective stand-alone treatment for some forms of anxiety. At the same time, it's quite common to become anxious about the thing that can help with anxiety, your athletic life. Athletic anxiety can manifest itself both generally and acutely.

In a general sense, think of athletic anxiety as low-grade constant worry: Am I training hard enough? Am I eating right? Am I dedicated enough? Tough enough? As with general anxiety in everyday life, athletic anxiety in this sense can lead to thoughts and behaviors that worsen the situation. You might interpret fatigue the day after a tough workout as evidence that you're in horrible shape, ramp up your training, and wind up that much more fatigued. Then, when you start to dread workouts or cut them short or go slower than you think you should, you attribute this state to being a wimp, rather than a clear sign from your body that it needs rest. And down the rabbit hole of self-doubt you go.

In an acute sense, anxiety over a race or a tough workout can become self-fulfilling. My current main running partner consistently underperformed in college meets because of angst over letting down her teammates. When things got tough during a race—as they almost always do—she worried about having to explain a poor result to her teammates. Doing so, of course, detracted from the task at hand, competing to the best of her ability on the day, and led to the subpar outcome she feared. Similarly, while prerace nerves are common, and understandable, they can lead to any number of physical outcomes that hamper performance, such as poor sleep, unhelpful hormonal surges, and even vomiting.

CBD can help with both forms.

Andrew Talansky started taking CBD in 2017, the year that the Tour de France veteran left cycling to become a professional Ironman triathlete. "One reason I was interested in CBD was that I was looking for help with the stress of transitioning into a new sport," he says. "I felt like it took the edge off at a time when I was really feeling the stress of launching a new career." Within a couple of weeks of taking a daily 25-milligram capsule, Talansky found he was less anxious during the day and therefore better able to focus on what needed to be done to become world-class in his new sport.

Talansky's fellow former pro cyclist Floyd Landis, who was stripped of his 2006 Tour de France title for doping, says that CBD has eased the transition to his new athletic life. (It's helped so much, in fact, that he founded his CBD company, Floyd's of Leadville.) While Landis no longer has high competitive goals, he still does hours-long rides and has had trouble balancing his old mindset with his current reality.

"One of the ways CBD has helped me the most is with being addicted, for lack of a better word, to endurance sports," he says. "You can feel like you should always be trying harder and training more, but sometimes what you really should be doing is laying down and relaxing and letting the work you've already done manifest itself. Over and above the anti-inflammatory effect and pain management effect, CBD has a calming effect for me that helps me let things go."

In this context, it makes sense that many of Landis's customers are middle-aged athletes, who must constantly assess the right mix of striving and backing off. This idea of CBD helping with acceptance, of coming to terms with new circumstances, strikes a chord with Aliffe.

"When I talk to people about cannabinoids, I talk about how they can change your perspective," he says. "People have a tendency to mechanize things—the human body is seen as a machine. People think if they grew up in one place with one profession, and then move to a wholly different environment, that life will continue the same way. They don't imagine how the difference in climate and culture will affect their outlook, how it will affect them socially, sexually, their appetite, their mental state. The body needs to adapt—it's different running a biological organism in London than it is in Jamaica. The endocannabinoid system needs to be able to manage what's going on, and cannabis can help make that happen."

Overall lessening of athletic anxiety should help training and competing on a day-to-day basis, as Talansky has experienced. There's also reason to think CBD can help with task-specific sport angst. "CBD can help with performance anxiety, because of its calming effect," says Michael Lewis, MD. "The result is better focus, better concentration, being calmer under fire."

Some strong evidence for this claim comes, admittedly, from outside the sporting world. Then again, what's a little athletic angst compared to public speaking?

In a series of experiments, Brazilian researchers tested whether a single dose of CBD lowered anxiety about speaking in public. Given that public speaking regularly ranks as people's top fear, even more than the fear of death, there's no better real-world task to use as a barometer of anxiety.

Their first study found that, when people with social phobia took CBD 90 minutes before a simulated public-speaking test, they experienced significantly reduced anxiety, cognitive impairment, and discomfort while speaking. After taking CBD, they were no more anxious than public-speaking subjects without social phobia. Subsequent studies found that CBD produced the same significant reduction in anxiety before public speaking by people without social phobia.

Most of us can picture times when, athletically, our bodies and minds aren't on the same page and drift farther apart the more we focus on getting things right. These are the sporting analogues to the negative self-talk many people experience during public speaking. ("Why did you just say that? You're rambling—get back on point! Stop thinking about your thoughts and just talk! This is going horribly." And so on.) University of Arizona researchers are investigating whether CBD can be equally helpful in golfers with the yips, which are typically described as a sudden and inexplicable decrease in fine motor skills during competition. The classic example of the yips is failing at what should be easy putts.

Although there are as many theories on what causes the yips as there are golfers, it's widely accepted that anxiety underlies the problem. If so, there's good reason to think that CBD will be found to be helpful. If you experience your own workout or competition version of the yips, try experimenting with various amounts of CBD in the hour or so before you might feel most anxious.

Cannabinoids and Exercise Euphoria

Let's be honest: some workouts just plain suck. With experience, you learn how to coax yourself through them. Some workouts are just sort of there, neither memorably bad nor Instagram-worthy good. These you complete on autopilot. And some workouts are peak physical and mental experiences. These you live for.

Despite being called "the runner's high," this fantastic phenomenon occurs in most forms of exercise, especially aerobic ones. It's more a you-know-it-when-it's-happening sensation than something that's strictly defined. Common subjective reports include feeling outside of time, feeling no discomfort, feeling in touch with something greater than one's self, and experiencing euphoria, a deep sense of well-being, and a lack of anxiety.

An exercise high's ineffable qualities and unpredictability make it hard to study in a lab. Most people attribute it to endorphins, the body's natural form of opioids. Endorphins are definitely part of the picture. A seminal German study used PET scans to image triathletes' brains during a two-hour run. Endorphin levels increased dramatically in the areas of the brain associated with mood, and these increases aligned with the triathletes' reports of euphoria.

But endorphins aren't the whole story. Other feel-good brain chemicals circulate in greater amounts during exercise, including endocannabinoids. David Raichlen, PhD, a professor of anthropology at the University of Arizona, has done interesting research on the intersection of endocannabinoids, exercise, and mood. In one study, he measured endocannabinoid levels before and after humans, dogs, and ferrets ran for 30 minutes on a treadmill (alas, not at the same time). Raichlen compared these findings to when the humans and dogs walked for 30 minutes on a treadmill and the ferrets sat quietly in a cage for half an hour. (He was unable to get the ferrets to walk consistently on the treadmill, so he had to improvise this control variable.)

After running, but not after walking, the humans' and dogs' endocannabinoid levels were significantly higher. This finding supports the idea that our endocannabinoid systems evolved to respond to the ancestral need for foraging and persistence hunting. Raichlen and others speculate that the benefit of increased endocannabinoid activity during activity is twofold. First, it provides temporary pain relief, which allows continued movement at a high enough speed to catch prey. Second, it provides a psychological reward (the feel-good aspect), which motivates a behavior that, for hunter/ gatherers, is "expensive" in terms of energy expenditure. The findings on dogs and ferrets strengthen this argument, because dogs also run to get food, but ferrets don't.

Further support for the endocannabinoid system's role in exercise euphoria came from a German study published in 2015. It found that mice who were given free rein to a running wheel were, in the aftermath of a run, less anxious and had greater pain tolerance than mice who were forced to be sedentary. That's about as close as possible to simulating the runner's high in mice because, as the researchers put it, "euphoria cannot be studied in mouse models."

To further investigate the link between the endocannabinoid system and runner's high, the researchers did the experiments twice more. First, they administered cannabinoid agonists (blocking agents) to the running mice. In that condition, the running mice were just as anxious and pain-sensitive as the sedentary mice. Second, the researchers genetically engineered some mice to not respond to endocannabinoid receptors. Here, too, the running mice lost their anxiety and their pain tolerance edge over sedentary mice. Therefore, the researchers concluded, the endocannabinoid system plays a key role in an exercise high.

What does all of this have to do with CBD? Well, if exercise temporarily boosts your endocannabinoid levels, then it's logical to wonder whether exogenous cannabinoids, such as a preworkout dropper of a CBD tincture, will affect that process.

Raichlen is considering conducting research on the interplay between CBD and exercise-influenced endocannabinoid levels. "One thing missing as people start using it more is how it affects the neurobiological rewards generally

associated with exercise," he says. "Does use of CBD enhance these effects, impair these effects, or have no media-
tion effect at all? Either way, this would be good to know."

When I offered the theory that CBD's known sedative
properties might blunt a runner's high, he replied, "This is
certainly a possibility. I suppose there's also the possibility
it could enhance the effects under certain circumstances."

Justin Young, who heads product development for
Floyd's of Leadville, ran competitively in high school and
college, and says, "I'm very familiar with getting that euphoria on 1 out of 10 runs, and always looking for it. I
would think using CBD before a workout would turn off a
runner's high more than trigger it. That's kind of the whole
point about CBD—this a cellular modulator that's keeping
your body from hitting extremes." The thinking here is a
more minor (and healthier) version of using CBD to come
down from a too-intense marijuana high.

It might come down to what exercise alone tends to do
for you physically and psychologically in the short term.

As I found while researching a previous book, *Running
Is My Therapy,* many people with anxiety prize exercise's
power to provide calm. For these people, it's reasonable to
think that pre-exercise CBD could accentuate that effect.
Avery Collins, a champion ultramarathoner from Steam-
boat Springs, Colorado, takes CBD oil and capsules when
he wakes—he calls it "my morning coffee"—to set himself
up for the long, challenging trail runs that are key to his
success.

Then there are people like me, whose normal state leans
toward the lethargic and who therefore appreciate how exercise energizes us. There's a good reason that some people

call this "activation"—during and after most runs, I feel like circuits in my body and brain are working with new vigor. I think of the difference as that between the weak internet connection my computer gets on an interstate bus and the download speed when I'm in a corporate office.

I experimented enough with prerun CBD to decide it detracted from rather than enhanced most runs. Not that I felt horrible running within an hour of a dose; I just didn't feel that spark and pop a few miles into a run as often. I now take CBD before a run in only one situation: if I'm doing a long run with a group and am stressing about being able to keep up and/or go the distance. A small amount of CBD on these mornings helps to calm the anxiety I feel when I wake, and I'm able to assure myself that the looming run, like 99 percent of those in the last four decades, will be fine once I'm in motion.

How to Maximize CBD's Help with Athletic Anxiety

By working out regularly, you're already doing one of the best things to combat anxiety. Here are some other ways to boost CBD's aid in lowering sport-specific anxiety.

Evaluate your attitude toward your sports and workouts:
If much of what you do in your athletic life is geared toward pleasing others, anxiety is inevitable. Will you measure up? What will they think of you if you don't meet their expectations? These worries often become self-fulfilling because they detract from your performance.

Most of us have why-am-I-doing-this moments in workouts and competitions. The key to overriding those doubts is having a convincing answer. And the key to answering convincingly is having personally meaningful goals. Regularly evaluate your athletic goals and the means to reach those goals, and make sure that you're the one in charge.

Consider whether you really need to get psyched up:
Before competitions or key workouts, many athletes turn to pump-up music and other aids to getting energized. Such practices might be counterproductive if you're naturally anxious in these situations. Try different warm-up routines to find one that prepares your muscles and mind without sending your adrenaline levels skyward.

When possible, exercise in a pleasant environment:
A growing body of research supports the idea of "green exercise," or working out in nature. People usually report a bigger mood boost and drop in anxiety after doing so. Water views have been found to provide a bonus amount of calm.

Green exercise doesn't necessarily mean deep in the woods. In a study conducted in Edinburgh, Scotland, brain activity associated with frustration, engagement, and long-term arousal fell, and activity associated with meditation rose, when the participants walked for just eight minutes in a small urban park.

If you're primarily an indoor exerciser, you can still seek to make your workout environment as nonstressful as possible. Choose a gym where you feel welcome and where the volume and visuals are in line with your preferences.

Don't feel that you have to push in every workout:
Constantly trying to outdo previous performances usually stalls your progress. Gains in most sports come from consistency and mixing harder and easier workouts. A variety of intensities is also helpful in addressing anxiety.

In a separate experiment from the one involving humans, dogs, and ferrets, David Raichlen measured endocannabinoid levels before and after people did 30-minute treadmill workouts at four intensities: very easy (walking for the study participants), light (jogging pace), moderate (standard conversational running pace), and very hard (close to 5K race pace for many of the participants). Only at the light and moderate intensities did the participants' endocannabinoid levels rise significantly.

Of course, there's more to a better mood than your levels of certain brain chemicals. You've probably felt enormous stress relief at times from pounding out a really hard workout. The relevant takeaway here is that lowered anxiety can often come from among your more moderate sessions.

Feel free to experiment:
Doing the same thing again and again can be comforting. In my sport, many runners have a few favorite loops that they regularly train on. Familiarity allows them to run on autopilot.

But repetition can also become a chore, especially when you constantly compare results from one day to the next. You might find yourself dreading workouts, or anxious during them, if you're worried about matching last week's time or number of reps. When this happens, remember that there are an infinite number of possible workouts you can do, and almost all will make you fitter. Top athletes regularly vary their workouts, partly to provide a slightly different stimulus and partly to avoid constant comparison. If it feels as if you're working hard, you are.

Think about technique, but not too often:
What do you think about when you exercise? It used to be said that accomplished athletes practice associative thinking (focusing on their technique, pace, bodily sensations, etc.), while more casual athletes use dissociative thinking (planning dinner, looking at the scenery, or doing anything else to take their minds off what they're doing).

It's now known that this model is overly simplistic. Most people use a mix of association and dissociation. The people who seem to always get the most out of themselves psychologically are adept at knowing which thinking strategies are best in a given situation.

Sometimes focusing on your technique is the best choice. For example, if you're floundering in the pool, or tiring on a run, a few simple cues to improve your form can work magic. They'll make your movements more efficient, which will reduce the amount of unnecessary energy you're expending, and they'll give you something to think about besides your fatigue.

But fixating on your form can cause your anxiety to spike, as any of the golfers in the yips-and-CBD study mentioned above can confirm. Monitoring your every movement can set off a cyclone of thoughts—and thoughts about thoughts—that hurt your performance. Research in this area suggests an optimal approach: Do an occasional body and technique scan, to make sure you're moving as efficiently as possible. Then refocus on other matters, such as completing the next segment of your workout or, yes, the scenery.

Remember, it's just sports:

Sports and athletic hobbies can provide meaning and purpose to how we live day to day. Regular exercise is integral to our physical and mental health and often is a key component of our social lives.

At the same time, it's just sports. Most of us make our living elsewhere. For everyone, our performance on the field or in the pool isn't the summation of our self-worth. There will be setbacks and shortfalls, and that's okay.

"In the grand scheme of things, sports are a safe space to fail," says Molly Huddle, a two-time track Olympian who holds the American record for 10 kilometers and the half marathon. "Those few hard losses are uncomfortable, but they help condition that fear of imperfection."

Relax and enjoy your athletic life. Don't you have enough to worry about elsewhere?

Key Points on CBD and Athletic Anxiety

- Anxiety often stems from a malfunction of the body's stress response system.
- The endocannabinoid system plays a key role in managing acute and chronic stress.
- Research suggests CBD can boost the endocannabinoid system's effectiveness at managing stress.
- CBD can help to reduce general anxiety about training and competition as well as anxiety about specific athletic performances.

Chapter 8

The Future of CBD

The CBD landscape has changed dramatically just in the last couple of years. Branding used to feature hemp leaves, tie-dye hues, and stoner puns. Now you see clean design and wellness-oriented wording. Product types have followed this evolution away from a close association with marijuana. CBD user demographics have quickly come to mirror those of overall society, including, of course, dedicated exercisers of all ages.

The passage of the 2018 farm bill, which legalized the cultivation of hemp at the federal level, will likely accelerate CBD's entry into everyday life. That development, in turn, should spur more changes in product type, manufacturing, price, point of sale, research, and more.

What will CBD, especially CBD for athletes, look like next year, in two years, in five years? "Everything is unknown in the world of the *Cannabis sativa* plant," deadpans Tom Adams, managing director and principal analyst for the consumer cannabis research firm BDS Analytics. Still, it's fun to speculate. With insights from Adams and other industry insiders, here's how the near future of CBD might play out.

What Will the FDA Do, and When?

When I started talking with CBD insiders in the summer of 2018, everyone said that once the new farm bill legalized hemp, the floodgates would open. CBD's legal status at the federal level would be unambiguous, and it would soon appear in mainstream outlets throughout the United States.

That didn't happen. President Trump signed the 2018 farm bill into law on December 20, 2018. Within hours, Scott Gottlieb, then the head of the Food and Drug Administration, issued a statement on CBD. The gist: CBD is a food additive, and the FDA has to approve any food additive before it can be sold in interstate commerce. Until that happens, most national chains will likely stay on the sidelines for fear of running afoul of the federal government.

"People without FDA experience might have assumed it was going to be smooth sailing as soon as the farm bill passed," Adams says. "That was never going to be the case because that's not how the FDA works. They take their job of being in charge of human health and safety very seriously."

If anything, the CBD market became more constricted. Some state and city health departments interpreted the FDA statement as new guidance on some CBD product types. In January, restaurants in New York City were told to stop adding CBD to cookies, coffee, and the like. Maine's health agency took "food additive" to mean anything consumed. It ordered retailers to pull from their shelves not only edibles like gummy bears but also tinctures and capsules, while allowing continued sales of vaping products and topicals. Illustrating the confusion around the matter, Maine's governor signed a law two months later that reinstated sales of the items that had been ordered removed. As this book went to the printer, CBD's status in individual states continued to vary to a potentially befuddling degree.

In March, CVS started carrying CBD products made by the cannabis brand Curaleaf in 800 of its 10,000 US stores. But CVS began only with topicals. It didn't immediately carry tinctures, capsules, and other product types that could be said to fall under the FDA's food-additive restriction. Around the same time, a spokesman for Whole Foods, which would seem to be an obvious CBD retailer, said, "Whole Foods Market will not sell products containing CBD until all issues regarding the regulatory status are completely resolved to our satisfaction."

To step back just a bit: federal law prohibits interstate commerce or marketing of something as a food or dietary supplement if it contains an ingredient that was the subject of clinical investigations or was sold as a drug before being marketed as a food or dietary supplement. The FDA's position is that CBD falls under this prohibition because CBD was approved as an ingredient in the epilepsy drug Epidiolex before it was marketed as a food. The FDA says the federal legalization of hemp doesn't change that underlying prohibition. "The FDA has its own processes and time lines, which are not the same as those of people who want to get it sorted out right now," Adams says. "In its role of protecting public health, the FDA has also taken the position, 'We don't care if this harms your business plan. We're the federal government.'"

At the same time, Gottlieb signaled that the FDA wanted to find a way to make this all work. "It wasn't 'We're about to shut you all down,'" Adams says. "It was 'Great, the farm bill has passed. Now come to us for approval.'"

CBD's ambiguous identity—Is it medicine? Is it food?—doesn't fit neatly into traditional FDA processes. That's why, in his December statement, Gottlieb spoke of "pathways available for those who seek to lawfully introduce these products into interstate commerce." He later expounded on that idea in February testimony before Congress.

"We're planning to seek broad public input on this pathway, including information on the science and safety behind CBD. But we know that this process could take time," Gottlieb said. "So we're also interested in hearing from stakeholders and talking to Congress on possible alternative approaches to make sure that we have an appropriately efficient and predictable regulatory framework for regulating CBD products."

There is a sort-of precedent for the FDA to go by here. You can go to any pharmacy and buy over-the-counter omega-3 fish oil supplements. Or, if you have extraordinarily high triglyceride levels, you can get an omega-3 prescription medicine. The same general product is sold as a supplement and a medication. In the case of omega-3, it was widely sold as a supplement before receiving FDA approval as a medication. That's the opposite time line of what the FDA says is the case with CBD. Still, this isn't entirely new ground for the FDA.

Gottlieb told lawmakers that CBD was one of his top priorities. Many interpreted "possible alternative approaches" to mean federal legislation. It looked as if CBD's remaining gray areas would soon be clarified. Then, in

March, Gottlieb resigned. Confusion and uncertainty about the near future again spiked. Before departing, Gottlieb announced an FDA stakeholders' meeting on the overall topic of CBD as a food additive. The meeting is more likely the first step in a long process than a quick journey to resolution.

If leadership change at the FDA stalls progress on CBD for too long, Congress could very well step in to settle the matter. Senate majority leader Mitch McConnell is from Kentucky, a leading state for growing hemp. House speaker Nancy Pelosi is from California, a leading state in the overall cannabis market. Support for the CBD industry is a rare area of bipartisan agreement.

"I think the cat's out of the bag way too much now," says Riley Cote, founder of BodyChek Wellness. "There's too much money, too many companies in this space. You can't push it all the way back in."

"We're still heading to the same place" of CBD being available nationwide in mainstream outlets, Adams says. "The process for getting approval for a food additive is much shorter than it is for a pharmaceutical. It may not be by the summer of 2019, but it will happen."

Where Will You Buy CBD?

Most CBD sales still take place online. The most common retail locations remain vape/smoke shops. That's slowly changing. If you visited me in Portland, Maine, you could buy one brand's CBD recovery drink powder at the local bike shop, and tinctures and creams by other brands at the nearby health food store.

But what about the Whole Foods and CVS that are within a short drive of those two stores? For CBD to become the daily-life fixture people predict, it will need to be widely available in mainstream outlets. When will that happen?

Well, to requote industry analyst Adams, everything is unknown in the world of the *Cannabis sativa* plant. The big sticking point for retail is the uncertainty over FDA regulations pertaining to CBD as a food additive. Until those regulations, a large national chain is unlikely to risk taking on the federal government just to sell CBD. Even if clarity from the FDA had immediately followed passage of the 2018 farm bill, however, there's disagreement about when national chains would have started selling CBD, and whose brands they would carry.

"Large corporations are risk-averse," says Kemal Whyte, founder of Grassroots Harvest. "A place like Whole Foods will start by carrying smaller companies' products rather than offer their own, and they'll see if it's worth doing their own thing." Michael Tatz, founder of the athlete-focused brand Resilience, agrees. "It's not easy to get into this business on a large scale," he says. "The supply chain and logistics are difficult. Easier risk management is to bring in reputable brands. Think about it: there's not a Whole Foods craft beer or kombucha."

Bob Bell, the owner of Floyd's of Leadville, says that the raw material for CBD, hemp, is another reason that national chains can't launch house brands overnight, despite how lucrative the CBD market is forecast to be.

"The real issue with big players is that you can't manufacture CBD in a perfect environment like you can for a synthetic pill," Bell says. "You still have to grow a plant, and that entails variables that you don't have with a lab, especially with climate change causing increasingly weird weather."

To Bell's point: It's relatively straightforward for a Whole Foods or CVS to offer a house brand of vitamin C and to have each pill contain the claimed amount of milligrams. But think about buying something like carrots—you know they'll be high in vitamin A but expect variability from one plant to the next. It would be much more cumbersome for a large corporation to efficiently produce a carrot-based product that is reliably consistent in its ingredients and amount of vitamin A.

"Big brands having their own product on a large scale is five to ten years away," Bell says.

Adams disagrees. "I suspect a major chain, somebody like CVS, will get a house brand of CBD through the FDA process before carrying other brands," he says. "The little mom-and-pop CBD product makers that have been in charge of the business don't have the resources to go through the FDA approval process for a food additive. The major corporations do. One will want to get their product out there first and own that market segment."

Will CBD Always Cost So Much?

One of the biggest barriers to CBD's popularity is its price. A high-quality, medium-potency one-ounce tincture typically costs between $50 and $90. If you were to take one dropper per day, you'd spend at least several hundred dollars a year. That's arguably a bargain if you see widespread benefits. But most of us devote most of our money to non-negotiable items. Regular CBD use is currently a financial stretch for a lot of people, even those who believe in it.

"The cost for me is prohibitive," says CrossFit competitor and coach Chase Knight. "My wife and I get by month to month. I don't think the prices are unreasonable, given the quality, but I have to prioritize. At this point for me, CBD is a luxury for that next level in training."

Floyd's of Leadville founder Floyd Landis expects average prices to fall by 10 to 20 percent over the next couple of years. Like others, he bases this prediction on simple economic supply and demand—not for CBD per se but for the hemp it's made from.

"Right now there's a premium being charged because it's a relatively new market and there's a lot of belief that there's a shortage of supply," Landis says. But in the wake of the 2018 farm bill, a lot more farmers are expected to start growing hemp. "In Kentucky, of 1,000 applicants to grow hemp in 2019, 98 percent of them are growing it for CBD," says Cote of BodyChek Wellness. "In late 2019, the market could be saturated with raw product." Cote and others say that dramatic increase in the supply of hemp should lead to lower CBD prices by the beginning of 2020 and that those new, lower prices will be the norm for the next couple of years. Cote says that by 2021 a tincture that now costs $80 will sell for $40 to $50.

"Hemp is very easy to grow if you're in the right environment and don't have high real estate costs," Landis says. "In places like Kentucky and Oregon, this stuff grows on its own." Cote adds that overseas growers with lower overhead costs will affect the US hemp market. "Business is business, and most of these companies will be sourcing the highest-quality but cheapest hemp they can find," Cote says. "It's a commodity like anything else."

Another major cost in producing CBD is the manufacturing process. Most experts expect the extraction and distillation of CBD (and in the case of full-spectrum products, other parts of the hemp plant) to remain expensive for now. "Any price drop in the near future is unlikely to be from advances in manufacturing," says Whyte of Grassroots Harvest. "That takes research and development, and it takes time to earn that investment back and get it to the consumer at a better price."

What Types of CBD Products Will Be Available?

We're in the midst of an explosion of new CBD products as brands seek to distinguish themselves from the hundreds of others that offer the standard tinctures, capsules, and creams.

Case in point: When I talked to him just after New Year's Day 2019, Don McLaughlin, the president of Pure-Power Botanicals, said, "I wouldn't be surprised to see CBD mixed into bedtime drinks." The following week, Steve Marchi, who runs the CBD Marketplace site, told me, "As of right now, I haven't seen a water-soluble, full-spectrum drink powder. Expect to see innovation around that." Guess what was introduced the following month? The "pot cocoa" I mentioned in Chapter 2, a water-soluble, full-spectrum powder designed to be consumed soon before sleep, created via a partnership between the brands Oleo and Elixinol. Other brands' full-spectrum, water-soluble drink powders have since become available, such as an electrolyte drink mix by the brand Arcanum.

"In terms of product type, I think the serious innovation will be in how to get CBD into regular consumer products," Marchi says. "Capsules are popular because people are familiar with the form—taking a CBD capsule is a natural transition if you're used to taking vitamins and other supplements. But I don't know that the oils will remain as popular. It's hard to see lots of people starting a new daily practice of placing things under their tongue. By the end of 2020, I would expect to see a lot of energy bars, drink mixes, and portable drinks."

Industry analyst Adams agrees, pointing to sports drinks as an obvious choice for brands targeting athletes and other busy, active people. "CBD is at least as useful as electrolytes and other things that are put into all sorts of products," he says.

Growth in everyday products should hasten a divergence that's already happening, according to McLaughlin. "The market is settling into two types of products. There's the type promising immediate benefits, analogous to asthma-relief delivery systems. That's vaping, tinctures with higher and higher doses of CBD, drink mixes, edibles. Then there's treating it like a nutritional supplement that you make a part of your everyday life to boost your overall health."

In Chapter 2, we saw that companies like McLaughlin's are integrating CBD into traditional herbal supplement formulations—St. John's wort for mood, chamomile and valerian for sleep, turmeric for inflammation, and so on. Look for this trend to continue and become even more fine-tuned.

The second aspect of the next generation of CBD products has to do with manufacturing. The main goal in this regard will be to increase the bioavailability of CBD in whatever form you take it. To date, most efforts have focused on getting the fat-soluble CBD molecule through the mostly-water environment of your body.

Another approach is being pursued by a biotech company started by Scott Palmer, MD, a team physician for the Chicago Bulls and Chicago White Sox. Palmer is beta-testing a topical cream that, instead of CBD, contains a cannabinoid derivative. The derivative binds magnesium (a biological metal) with cannabidiolic acid, or CBDa. What's the difference?

"Plants do not make CBD or THC," Palmer says. "They make the acid form of these cannabinoids. The conversion to CBD and THC occurs during drying or processing the plant." According to Palmer, cannabinoids are excellent coordinators of metals, and the metals, in turn, improve the efficacy of the cannabinoids. "Our product appears to be about 1,000 times as strong as CBD in all sorts of models," he says.

I had the opportunity to try Palmer's topical cream. Bearing in mind all the necessary caveats about experiments of one, I found it to be noticeably more effective than the many other CBD-related topicals I've used. While working on this book, my running primarily occurred on snowy, icy, slanted roads during the Maine winter. The poor footing aggravated where my left vastus lateralis, a quadriceps muscle, attaches to the knee. The vastus lateralis acts as a knee extensor, which in running involves bringing your lower leg through a full range of motion in the back kick portion of the gait. Being unable to run with my normal form made the already-challenging winter conditions that much more troublesome. I developed a series of compensatory aches elsewhere on both legs.

For two months I got little relief from targeted foam rolling, icing, stretching, strengthening, and topical CBD application. All it took was one treacherous run to undo whatever progress I made. Within two days of applying Palmer's cream twice a day to the vastus lateralis insertion area, I began to notice significant improvement, and within a week the stiffness and tenderness I'd felt there was gone. Once that problem was fixed, the aches elsewhere also disappeared.

I offer this anecdote not to promote Palmer but to say that it's an exciting time to be an athlete who uses CBD. Palmer's company is also developing an oral form of its CBDa-magnesium product. Existing brands continue to investigate how to increase bioavailability. Those of us who already feel that we benefit from incorporating CBD into our regimes should soon see that much more benefit.

CBD is here to stay, and is likely to become more effective, more accepted, more available, and less expensive. I hope this book has helped you decide whether CBD has a place in your life.

Key Points About the Future of CBD

- National grocery and pharmacy chains are eager to carry CBD products but are waiting on the Food and Drug Administration to resolve regulatory issues before really jumping in.
- Prices will probably go down by 10 to 20 percent in the next couple of years.
- Product development will center on integrating CBD into more everyday food and drinks and increasing the bioavailability of CBD in current products.

Glossary

Bioavailability: How much of the CBD in a product your body absorbs. Most CBD products have low bioavailability because the CBD molecule resists being absorbed in the body's mostly water environment. Increasing bioavailability is a top goal for next-generation CBD products.

Cannabinoid: A chemical compound that binds to cellular receptors in your body. Cannabinoids are produced inside your body (endocannabinoids), by plants (exogenous cannabinoids), or in a lab (synthetic cannabinoids). CBD and THC are the two most prevalent cannabinoids in the cannabis plant.

Cannabinoid receptors: Structures on the surface of cells throughout your body. When activated by cannabinoids, the receptors cause cellular changes in the organs they're associated with.

Cannabis: The plant from which CBD is extracted. A cannabis plant is classified as hemp if it contains no more than 0.3 percent THC. Marijuana is a cannabis plant with more than that amount of THC. The CBD products discussed in this book are made from hemp.

Cannabidiol/ CBD: One of the cannabinoids found in the cannabis plant. CBD products made from hemp are nonintoxicating, legal, and safe to consume.

Endocannabinoid system: The cannabinoid receptors and cannabinoids produced by your body. The endocannabinoid system is thought to regulate most other bodily systems and to be responsible for maintaining balance among those systems. CBD is believed to improve the functioning of the endocannabinoid system.

Entourage effect: The claim that full-spectrum CBD products are more efficacious than CBD isolate products. The claim makes sense on a theoretical level but has yet to be backed by clinical research.

Full-spectrum: A product that contains many parts of the cannabis plant in addition to CBD. The components of full-spectrum products are said to work synergistically to produce the entourage effect. Full-spectrum hemp-derived CBD products are likely to contain trace amounts of THC.

Isolate: A product containing CBD but no other parts of the cannabis plant. CBD isolates are a good choice for people who don't want to consume the trace amounts of THC that can be in full-spectrum products.

Slow-wave sleep: The deepest phase of sleep, during which many bodily repairs happen. CBD can increase the amount of time spent in slow-wave sleep, thereby potentially speeding recovery.

Sublingual dosing: Taking an oral solution by placing it under your tongue and keeping it there for several seconds. Some people say taking CBD sublingually increases your body's absorption of CBD.

THC: Shorthand for tetrahydrocannabinol, the cannabinoid responsible for producing a marijuana high.

Topical: A cream, salve, balm, etc., applied to the skin. CBD topicals can be an effective way to treat site-specific pain and inflammation.

Purchasing Checklist

Here's a quick guide to what to look for when shopping for CBD. For more information about each criterion, see Chapter 3.

Make sure the product you're considering . . .

❑ **Clearly lists the ingredients**
Ingredients should be easy to find on the product label.

❑ **Uses only natural ingredients**
No artificial flavors, colors, or preservatives are needed for CBD to be effective.

❑ **Uses an extraction method that doesn't require solvents**
CO_2 extraction is the industry standard and most common, but you may see different methods that were developed for increased bioavailability. The important thing is that the extraction method is clearly stated and doesn't involve solvents.

❑ **Clearly states the potency**
The product should list how much CBD it contains,

either in the total package (as in tinctures and topical solutions) or per single serving (as in capsules).

❑ **Uses organic or at least non–GMO hemp grown in the USA**
Hemp grown in the United States is more likely to be cultivated with natural farming methods. *Consumer Reports* suggests looking for companies in states that have legalized the recreational and medical use of cannabis, "since they tend to have stricter standards."

❑ **Has been tested by a third party**
Results from third-party testing should be easy to find, via either a QR code on product packaging or the brand's website. Third-party testing should clearly show that the product contains the claimed amount of CBD and minimal to no THC.

❑ **Doesn't claim to cure or treat any disease**
Such claims are not allowed by the FDA. Also remember that CBD is not a magic bullet, and any company that presents it that way should be treated skeptically.

❑ **Is responsibly priced**
Beware of both suspiciously cheap and outrageously expensive products, and products that are sold through multilevel marketing or subscription services. Refer to the price range listed on page 73 for a rough estimate of how much each product should cost.

Acknowledgments

Thank you to everyone who allowed me to interview them for this book. I learned and benefited from every conversation. Brittany Confer, Steve Marchi, and Scott Palmer were especially generous with their time and knowledge.

Danielle Curtis and the rest of the Penguin Random House team enthusiastically supported the idea of a short book (produced in a short time) on CBD for athletes.

Brian Dalek of *Runner's World* indulged my initial journalistic interest in CBD and then allowed me to step aside from most of my *Runner's World* responsibilities while I worked on this book.

About the Author

Scott Douglas is a contributing writer for *Runner's World*. He has been published on health and fitness topics in the *Washington Post, The Atlantic,* and *Slate.* He is the author or coauthor of several other books, including *Running Is My Therapy, Advanced Marathoning,* and the *New York Times* best-sellers *26 Marathons* and *Meb for Mortals.* A resident of South Portland, Maine, Scott has run more than 100,000 miles in the last four decades.